In-Between Years
Life after a positive Huntington's disease test

Steven Beatty

Amazon Direct Publishing

Dedication

For Michelle. Your support has been never-ending, as is my love for you.

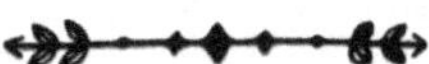

Also, for all the Huntington's disease research participants the world over. You are true Heroes. Thank you.

Contents

1. Introduction   1

2. My Huntington's Disease Story   3
   My Dad
   My Sisters

3. What is Huntington's Disease?   8
   The Beast
   Genetics
   Symptoms
   Treatment

4. What Does My CAG Number Tell Me?   12

5. Becoming Involved with With Huntington's Disease   16
   Associations
   Support groups and Chapters
   Fundraising and Awareness
   Education
   Conferences

6. Your Healthcare Team   23
   Healthcare Varies the World Over
   Geneticist
   Neurologist

Psychiatrist

Counsellor

Research team

7. Participating in Research   29

What is Enroll-HD?

Getting involved in Enroll-HD

Keeping up to date on research outcomes

8. Symptom Seeking   34

9. Fear   38

Fear of being a burden

Fear of not being there for my kids

Fear that my kids may have inherited the HD gene from me

Fear of the unknown

Fear that there won't be an effective treatment for my kids
if they need it

Fear that there won't be an effective treatment for me before
I'm lost

10. When Do I Tell People About My Huntington's Dis-   44
ease?

Work

Genetic Discrimination

Genetic Information Non-Discrimination Act (GINA)

Genetic Non-Discrimination Act (GNA)

Family and Friends

Dating

Children

11. Anger   51

Why Do We Feel Anger?

What Do We Do About It?

12. Making Babies   54
       Sperm or Egg Donation
       Prenatal Diagnosis (PD)
       Preimplantation Genetic Diagnosis (PGD) In-Vetro Fertil-
       ization (IVF)
       Non-Disclosure or Exclusion Testing
       Natural
       Adoption

13. Staying Positive   60
       Family and Friends
       Support from Other In-Betweeners
       Counselling
       Medications
       Exercise, and More Exercise
       Food for Positive Thought

14. Exercise   65
       What is Exercise Anyway?
       Exercise is Good for Your Psychological Health
       Exercise and Your Heart
       Be a Good Role Model

15. Caring   69
       Preventing Caregiver Burnout
       Seeing Our Future as we Care for HD Symptomatic Parents

16. Guilt   73
       What to Do About Guilt?

17. Journaling   76
       Smartphone Application
       Paper Journaling
       Video Journaling

Why Journal?

18. Planning Ahead   81
    Advanced Directives
    Insurance
    Bucket List
    Brain Donation

19. Following the Latest Developments in Huntington's   86
    Disease News
    HD Buzz
    Facebook Groups
    Association Newsletters and Chapter Meetings

20. Is Huntington's Disease Predictive Testing Even Worth   90
    the Trouble?
    Don't Rush into the Decision
    Once You Know, You Can't Un-Know
    Do I Have Any Regrets?

21. When Symptoms Start   93
    What does it mean to be symptomatic?
    What do we do if we think we're symptomatic?

22. I Look Forward to the Day When There Won't be a   97
    Need for this Book

23. Calls to Action and Conclusion   99
    Here are some calls to action for you to take away

About the Author   105

Chapter 1
Introduction

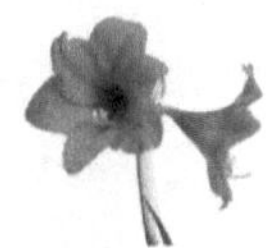

"It's not the result we were hoping for."

Those eight little words echoed in my head like a Mack Truck rolling through a tunnel. A Mack Truck in the form of a telephone call from a Genetic Counsellor at my local hospital.

"What, me?", was my gasped response.

"Yes," she replied, "I'm sorry."

I sat there in total stunned silence and started to think about all the consequences related to what she had just told me. What this news would mean for my family and me, possibly for generations to come.

That was the moment my life completely changed. Changed in pretty much almost every conceivable way. How I looked to the future. How I reflected on the past. How I coped with the present. It changed what I found to be important and what I saw not even to be worth my time.

It was the day I found out I was positive for the gene mutation that's responsible for Huntington's disease. The disease that I've heard some resources refer to as "one of the worst diseases you can get" and "it's like having Alzheimer's, ALS and Parkinson's disease all at the same time!"

Where was I to go from there? What was I supposed to do? How could I cope with the knowledge that, unless a sufficient treatment came along soon, this disease was going to kill me in the not too distant future?

I had no idea what to do next, and I felt utterly alone.

That's the reason behind why I've written this book. It's for those of us going through the "in-between years": the years following our HD genetic testing, but before the symptoms of the illness have begun to take hold. The years when we may struggle with this look into the crystal ball we've been given, for whatever reasons are personal to us. The years when we symptom-hunt and worry about every forgotten purse and each trip and stumble. The years when we watch and care for other Huntington's disease affected loved ones and wonder, how long until it's *our* turn.

It's during those in-between years that we may struggle the most.

Chapter 2

My Huntington's Disease Story

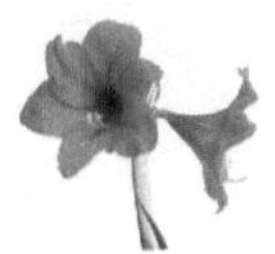

My Huntington's disease story begins like most people in the HD community: with a family history.

I inherited the gene mutation from my father. I'm not able to track it very far back in history, however, as its first arrival into my known genealogical tree was with my paternal grandmother, my father's mom. I say *known* because she was adopted and whatever happened in the genealogy before her is not information I'm able to access.

My memories of her are, unfortunately, not all that good. I only remember her being ill and living in a Psychiatric Hospital. In my mind, I can visualize her all scrunched up sitting in a chair and not interacting with anyone.

Perhaps, as a fellow in-betweener, you have similar memories of a grandparent.

At that time, my grandfather was living in a town about an hour from the hospital, and he would come up on the train every so often to visit her. Usually on Sundays, as I recall. It was during those visits that I would accompany the family to the hospital to see the scrunched up old lady I knew as "grandma."

My grandmother died in the early 1990's, before Huntington's disease genetic testing was possible. Even though that was the case, I distinctly remember that, within family discussions, her diagnosis seemed to be understood as being Huntington's disease. That's what I recall being told. I'm not sure what diagnosing criteria were used in her case. Being that she was adopted, it was quite likely that Huntington's disease had come into her life completely out of left field.

How terrifying that must have been for her and my grandfather.

My grandparents had five kids: four sons and a daughter. I wouldn't describe it as being an overly close family and, to be honest, I never really knew my dad's three brothers.

Two of my dad's brothers would eventually develop Huntington's disease themselves during the typical adult-onset period in their thirties and forties. Since I was not close to these uncles, their illness was not a part of my life. I did not watch them progress through their HD journey, I was never in the caregiving role for them, and there were no funerals or celebrations of life as far as I even knew.

They lived. They suffered through Huntington's disease. They died. And I played no role in any of it.

My Dad

My father, as it has turned out, has been a bit of an anomaly in our family as far as his Huntington's disease is concerned. In fact, I've spent much of my adult life under the impression that he was *negative* for the Huntington's disease gene mutation. That, of course, would mean that I was also negative.

In fact, he even told me years ago that he had been tested once the genetic testing for HD was available and received a negative result. This fact was, of course, not accurate.

I'm not sure why he decided to tell me that. Maybe it was his personality changing slowly with his HD, or perhaps he thought he was protecting me in some way, I don't know. And I can't get a straight answer out of him today.

Yes, that's right, I said *today*. My dad is still alive at age 69-years-old.

I'm not sure if my dad's HD is very slow in its progression, or if he has a late-onset form of the illness, but he has already outlived his two brothers by 15 years or so. Also, he is still living on his own and managing his affairs, but I can see that starting to slide.

That odd disease progression, combined with his lie about testing negative, lead me to spend the first 40 years of my life thinking I was not at risk of developing Huntington's disease.

No risk at all.

You could say ignorance is bliss, and I probably wouldn't argue with you, but it wasn't until that 41st year of mine that I started to question whether my dad was, in fact, negative for Huntington's disease.

I began to notice changes in him. I saw changes in his personality. De-conditioning in his muscles. Weight loss. I don't remember where I had the initial thought about HD, but I began to ask myself, *"is there such a thing as late-onset Huntington's disease?"*

I took to the computer and did some research. Sure enough, late-onset HD was a real thing, and it sounded a lot like how he was presenting to me.

I lost my breath. Right there in front of my computer. If you were looking at my face, it was likely quite pale.

Professionally, I work as a Registered Nurse, and I felt comfortable calling the local genetics clinic and referring myself. I proceeded to book an appointment to discuss the process and appropriateness of undergoing the testing process for HD. Once I was there, they were very supportive, and after hearing my explanation about why I thought it was reasonable for me to be tested, they agreed, and my blood was drawn that very same day.

The Geneticist seemed confident that the result would be negative and, quite frankly, so was I. To be honest, I barely even thought about it all that much over the five weeks I had to wait for the result. Again, ignorance was bliss.

So confident were we in a negative result, that the Genetic Counsellor and I agreed that the results could be given to me over the phone. I didn't have to schedule an appointment to go to the clinic in person. I didn't have to surround myself with support from loved ones. I would just take the call.

"It's not the result we were hoping for."

Tell me about it. My CAG repeat score was 42. *What does that even mean*? I was ignorant about the science behind HD. I had never really taken the time to learn about it.

Why would I? *I wasn't at risk*!

Once my result came back as being positive, I had to let everyone in the family know about the outcome, especially my two sisters. And my father for that matter, as he had not had a genetic test himself up to that point. I was breaking the news to him as well.

The genetic dominoes were tumbling.

My Sisters

My two sisters, aged 43- and 22-years-old at the time, were now faced with the decision that everyone at risk for HD faces: whether to proceed with the Huntington's disease genetic testing or not. Neither of them was having any symptoms at that point, but in the case of my older sister, she already had a 2-year-old child, my nephew, who would now be at risk if it turned out that she was carrying the mutated gene.

These are such difficult and personal decisions to make, and there will be more discussion about the testing process in subsequent sections of this book.

Both of my sisters decided to undergo the predictive genetic testing, and the results were split: the younger sister was negative, and the older sister was positive. My nephew *was* indeed now at risk.

More dominoes.

"Fuck," was my response, when my older sister reported her test result to me. What else are you even going to say? At the same time, I felt complete joy for my younger sister who turned out to be negative. My emotions were on a roller-coaster, and I hadn't yet even come to terms with my *own* diagnosis.

Talk about a complete shake-up of my family's whole world. In the matter of a couple of short months, we went from Huntington's disease not even being on the radar, to having me, my sister and my dad all positive for the gene mutation. Not to mention, my two kids and my nephew were now known to be at risk. They *each* have a 50 percent chance of inheriting this damn disease.

More dominoes placed at the end of the line. How will they fall?

Chapter 3

What is Huntington's Disease?

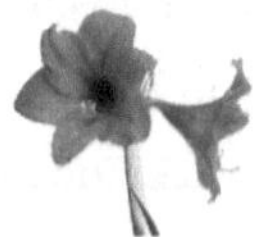

If you're reading this book, there's a good chance you already know a thing or two about Huntington's disease, so I won't rewrite an encyclopedia here. With that said, I do not doubt that someone newly introduced to the topic may be starving for information.

The whole point of this book is to learn how to cope with these in-between years. A great way to decrease the fear and anxiety associated with the entire thing is to learn more about the beast that is Huntington's disease.

Knowledge is power.

Knowledge gives you hope.

Knowledge allows you to take control.

Knowledge teaches you, "*holy shit, there is a lot of great research going on out there!*"

Following my positive genetic test, I *literally* read a textbook. Not every single word, but probably 80% of the bloody thing. It was this book here:

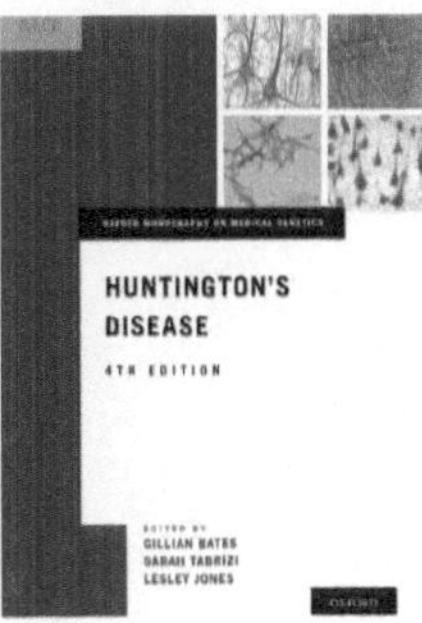

(Image:)

I soaked up the words in that book like a dry sponge soaking up water in a sink. I think my head actually made a slurping sound. I'm not suggesting that you must read a whole textbook, but for me, it helped me to develop that knowledge, which as I mentioned, can be so empowering.

The Beast

Huntington's disease is a neurodegenerative disease that affects parts of the brain and leads to behavioural, cognitive and movement disorder symptoms.

HD is caused by a mutation in a specific gene, now known as the Huntington gene. Everyone has this gene, but in people who will develop Huntington's disease, there's a part of the gene that repeats itself more than what's normal. That's the mutation, and that's what people are talking about when they mention "CAG repeats."

The "CAG" is the section that is repeating, and if the number of repeats passes a certain threshold, the person will develop Huntington's disease at some point in their life.

I'll talk more about CAG repeats in the next chapter. I think it's a topic those of us who are in the in-between years spend a lot of time thinking about because it can give clues as to when the disease might start to become symptomatic in a person's life.

Genetics

Huntington's disease is an autosomal dominant disorder (say what?!) which means that a person only needs one copy of the mutated gene to develop the disease (we get two, one from each parent). And what's worse, each child from someone who has the mutated HD gene themselves will have a 50 percent chance of inheriting the genetic disorder.

50/50. A coin toss. It's a heartbreaking thing. With that said, as we'll discuss in future chapters, science is helping us here. There are methods already out there to assist us with HD gene negative pregnancies.

Symptoms

Huntington's disease is usually described as affecting us in three different ways: movement, cognitive and psychiatric or behavioural symptoms. Each person's presentation with HD is unique. It's not unusual to see a little bit of everything in an HD patient, or, see someone whose symptoms are dominated by one disorder over the others.

There are more rare presentations of the condition, such as juvenile or late onset Huntington's disease, where symptoms can again be entirely different than what is seen with the more common adult-onset HD.

Treatment

At this point, there are no effective treatments for Huntington's disease itself. What this means is, there are treatments for specific symptoms, like medication to help decrease the chorea (movements) as an example, but for all intents and purposes, HD is a fatal disease with no cure.

Yet.

Like I said earlier, science is working itself to the bone (I know some scientists and it ain't pretty, they're all bony) on finding effective treatments for the disease itself and the future is bright.

One of the ways to be successful during these in-between years is to remember this fact, so I'll repeat it.

The future is bright!

As you read this, there are people in clinical studies testing new therapies! Right now! As we speak, err, uh, read!

Chapter 4

What Does My CAG Number Tell Me?

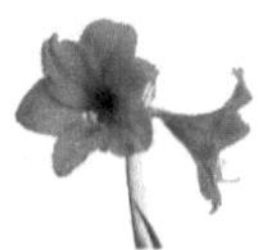

After my genetic counsellor broke the bad news about my positive Huntington's disease result in my predictive testing, she informed me that my "CAG repeat score" was 42.

42 repeats. As I mentioned in a previous chapter, at that point in time, I was still entirely ignorant about the science behind HD and, the number 42 meant nothing to me.

I quickly learned, however (remember the textbook?), that the number refers to how many times the gene repeats this cytosine-adenine-guanine (CAG) section of the DNA within the Huntington gene.

Everyone has the Huntington gene within them. And everyone has a section of CAG that repeats. It's only when the number of repeats passes a certain threshold that Huntington's disease will occur. Have a look at the following chart:

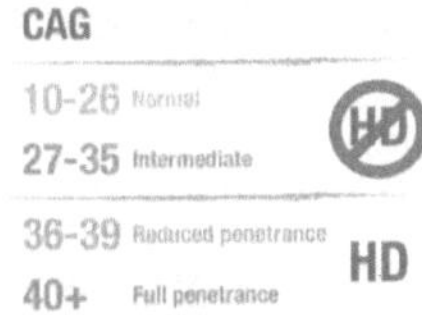

(Image:)

You can see that anything below 35 is considered a no HD zone. Then there's the gray area between 36–39 where a person *may* develop Huntington's disease later in life. Above 40 is the full HD zone. In other words, the "you're screwed zone."

Let's have a look at my predictive test result below:

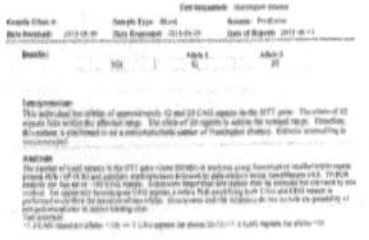

(Image: Steven Beatty)

You can see my 42 there, but I also have a 20 from my mother. That 20 is normal, but the 42 from my father puts me in the "you're screwed" zone of full HD penetrance.

This fact means that at some point in my life, I will develop Huntington's disease-related symptoms.

But *when*?

I think that has got to be the most commonly asked question for those of us in these in-between years:

"When will the cursed symptoms begin to take control of my life??"

Unfortunately, it's not an easy question to answer and there are a lot of unknowns, but again our dear friend science can provide some clues.

The data shows that, in general, the *higher* CAG repeat score you have, the *younger* you will be when symptoms develop.

I say "in general" because to see this correlation between CAG score and age of HD symptom onset; you need to look at a large sample of people.

Here's a scatter graph to show what I mean:

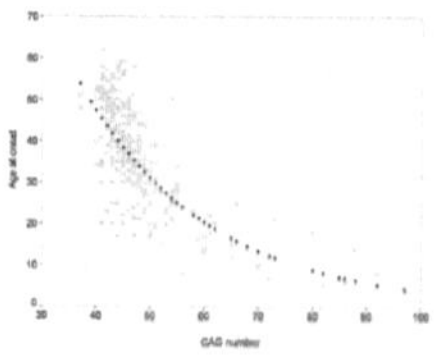

(Image:)

This graph plots 319 Huntington's disease patients. The numbers along the left side represent age at onset of symptoms, and the bottom number is the CAG repeat score. The relationship between CAG repeat and age of onset is quite clear, but what is also clear, is that there is still a great deal of variety and outliers there.

For example, let's look at my number of 42 repeats. Tracking that up, you can see some people had symptoms begin in their 20's, and others had symptoms start in their 50's.

The general trend and correlation are there, but for *individual* people, the CAG cannot be used to predict the age of symptom onset definitively.

Here's the data demonstrated in a chart:

(Image:)

In this chart, when using my good old 42 as an example, the median age of onset is 49-years-old. That, in no way, guarantees me an age of onset of 49. It's just the median when looking at the Data from a large group of people.

Let's remember my dad. His CAG repeat score is the same as mine: 42. And his age of onset was well above 49-years-old.

So, why the diversity?

There's a lot of research going on right now to try and answer that very question and the answer is probably multifaceted.

What role does exercise play in the age of onset of Huntington's disease symptoms? What other genetic traits or biomarkers might a person have that contributes? Science doesn't have the answers yet, but I have no doubt they will come.

Chapter 5

Becoming Involved with With Huntington's Disease Associations

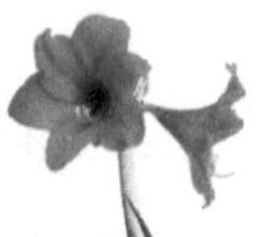

Following the positive result in my Huntington's disease predictive testing, not only was I hungry for knowledge, but I was also hungry to know that I wasn't alone.

I felt that way and, given the rarity of the disease, I imagine several of you in-betweeners have felt the same way.

I knew of no one in my local area who was part of a Huntington's disease family. My sister, who had also tested positive in her HD testing, lived hours away. Even in my career as a Registered Nurse working in the home care sector, I had never come across an HD "patient" in my work.

I felt completely alone.

When my Geneticist was getting me set up with a Neurologist (more on that in the next chapter), I was also given a package of information on the Huntington Society of Canada (HSC). In my part of the world, the HSC is the not-for-profit support and fundraising Association for HD families. There are similar Associations located in areas all around the world, such as the Huntington's Disease Society of America (HDSA) in the United States, and the Huntington's Disease Association (HDA) in the United Kingdom.

For me, becoming involved with the Huntington Society was the *single most rewarding and positive thing that I've done during these in-between years*. I understand that not everyone wants to get involved with groups. I acknowledge that genetic discrimination is a real thing and that HD positive individuals may decide to remain private. However, I do encourage you to consider reaching out. Let me explain why.

Support groups and Chapters

Along with fundraising, supporting Huntington's disease families is one of the core roles HD Associations serve; that goes without saying. Chapters are an excellent way for Associations to fulfill this task.

A "Chapter" is a group, usually situated in a specific geographical area, that is formed by an Association to serve and support people in that area. Chapters receive assistance from the Association's head office to run fundraising and education events within the area, and the Association may also provide healthcare professionals, such as Social Workers or Counsellors, to further assist the members and attend the Chapter meetings.

Chapter meetings are going to be planned differently depending on where you are in the world and what the needs of your group are.

Geography can play a crucial role here. Large population centres like cities may have regular meetings every month with structured outlines that work well for a larger group of people.

Let's use my fantastic mother as an example (oh, come on, she'll be so happy that I included her in here!). She lives in a large city and the Chapter meetings she attends usually flow like this:

- The group will meet to review the latest in Huntington's disease news.

- There may be a guest speaker to present a topic of interest or someone from the Association head office may be there to speak.

- They discuss their current and future fundraising activities and provide updates.

- Finally, the group splits into two: the HD affected individuals will move to another area to have a meeting with the social worker assigned to that geographical area. Family members and caregivers will group together to discuss issues and concerns related to their caregiving role.

This arrangement can be incredibly helpful for the in-betweeners there, especially early on in their HD journey, as they will quickly learn that they are not alone in their battle. They learn that other in-betweeners are sharing similar experiences and expressing similar concerns.

This set-up is also vital for the loved ones and caregivers present at the Chapter meeting as well. I discuss caregiver burnout in a future Chapter, but I will say here that being in a safe and private space to share concerns related to caregiving, without the HD member of the family present, can be very therapeutic.

At Chapter meetings, you may discover other members of the Huntington's disease community who are living very close by to where you are, and you may not even realize it. Being involved with a HD Association may be the only way you learn about each other and get that local support (if you want it, remember you're free to make your own decisions about how you manage your in-between years).

My mother's Chapter does a great job, but as I mentioned earlier, she lives in a large city (hi mom!). There are many Huntington's disease families and individuals that live in more rural areas, such as myself.

When I initially reached out to the Huntington Society following my test results, I quickly realized that there was no Chapter or support group anywhere near me. In fact, I was looking at about a two-hour drive to get to the nearest meeting, and who wants to do that on a Tuesday evening? Not me.

With that said, Huntington Society Associations do often organize events that are separate from Chapter meetings and reach out to larger geographical areas and populations. Education events and conferences are a good example, which I'll discuss in a moment.

Before moving on, however, I just wanted to touch on one other aspect as it relates to making contacts in the HD community. This is the age of the Internet!

The Internet has completely changed the way we find information and meet, virtually anyway, other like-minded people. This is no different in the HD community.

There are several online groups out there, on Facebook for example, where you can meet and interact with people from all over the world. This topic will be expanded on in a future chapter of this book.

My reason for bringing up the internet here is to mention that there are *virtual* Chapters connected with some HD Associations. Here's an example from the Huntington Society of Canada where there is a virtual Chapter for young people:

"Young People Affected by Huntington disease (YPAHD) is a virtual youth chapter of the Huntington Society of Canada and is open to all youth. YPAHD provides a community and support network for young people affected by Huntington disease5."

This is a great way to support the youth in our HD community who are often dealing with so much in their lives and, are often connected to the internet. They can reach out and support each other at almost any time via social media and other online services.

Fundraising and Awareness

As I mentioned above, fundraising is one of the key functions Huntington's disease Associations serve. It's such an important thing. Without fundraising initiatives, the Association and Chapters would not even exist. Often, an Association will split the fundraising money it brings in between family support services (such as supporting Chapters and events) and research.

It goes without saying that we want to see money, lots of money, going towards research. Lots and lots of money.

And, then more money.

Huntington's disease Association fundraising events are most often organized by individual Chapters to take place within their geographical area. For example, my mother's (hi mom, love ya!) Chapter runs a very successful hike event that brings in thousands of dollars every year. Local businesses act as corporate sponsors to fund tents and food and those logistical expenses. Participants collect individual sponsors to raise the cash.

And all that money is funneled directly into research and family support services. Split 50/50.

For those of us in the in-between years, participating in, and even organizing, fundraising events can be such a rewarding undertaking. The money raised is going right into the research that is going to cure Huntington's disease. It's going directly into supporting families and loved ones who are so often struggling in the caregiver role.

It's giving hope.

Education

Huntington's disease Associations will assist with HD education, again most often through Chapters, but occasionally through broad-er, conference type education events.

The associations are there to assist with literature, audio-video me-dia, internet streaming and guest speakers among other things.

Education events are another great way to meet and network with other members of the HD community, all while learning something new.

For people who do not live near a Chapter, but can attend the odd education event, these can be very beneficial. Furthermore, these types of events are often streamed live through the internet or saved online after the fact to watch later.

Conferences

At the beginning of this article, I confessed that becoming involved with my Huntington's disease Association was the most important thing I've done so far during these in-between years. As I mentioned, the support and peer development have been paramount in my ability to combat feelings of being alone in the HD battle.

This was never more obvious than when I attended my first National Conference.

Being surrounded and supported by dozens and dozens of other in-betweeners and Huntington's disease families, participating in education sessions and being brought up to date on all the latest HD research and news was priceless.

Speaking of priceless, conferences can be expensive. There is no doubt about that. Even more so if you live in a country that covers a large ground area and you need to include airline tickets into the cost. With that said, there may be a process through your Huntington's disease Association to apply for funding assistance to attend a national conference. Be sure to ask if you're thinking about attending.

Chapter 6
Your Healthcare Team

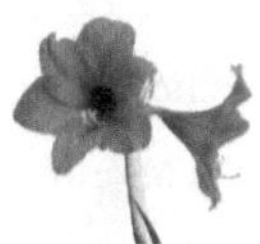

Having the support from a healthcare team that you trust is paramount during the in-between years. These are the professionals that you will grow to trust and who you will turn to with questions, concerns and guidance.

And, when HD related symptoms do begin to take hold, these are the people who will help treat you, support your caregivers and link you with research opportunities.

Healthcare Varies the World Over

Healthcare systems around the world are all unique, and it's beyond the scope of this article to break down the nitty-gritty details of each country. Undoubtedly, a mistake or two would be published which would be unfortunate.

The goal here is to provide an overview of the different healthcare professionals whom you may meet as you travel through these in-between years.

Geneticist

For me, the Geneticist was the first professional I encountered as it relates to my Huntington's disease journey.

This was where my HD predictive genetic testing and counselling took place and was the point where my life started going in a completely different direction.

The Geneticist's involvement is short: counsel and test. And counsel a bit more. It sounds so simple, but *wow*, the results can be so life-changing.

The counselling is there to help prepare and support you through the emotionally complicated process of being told that you have Huntington's disease. It's also there to inform you about issues you may not think about before being tested, such as genetic discrimination and insurance.

The knowledge and information you're given prior to the predictive test may even cause you to put the testing on hold. Perhaps you want to give more thought as to how a positive result may affect your acquisition of medical or life insurance in the future.

Most countries have some law in place to prevent genetic discrimination, but you need to know these things before the test so that you can make an informed decision.

Following the genetic counselling and predictive testing, the Geneticist's final task is to refer you on to a Neurologist. For me, I was done with the Genetics Clinic at that point, and I hope I never have to go back, quite frankly.

I hope my kids never have to go through that, which I suppose is wishful thinking. Let me rephrase that: I hope my kids can go through that knowing that there is an effective treatment for Huntington's disease if their predictive testing turns out to be positive.

Before moving on, I will say, the Geneticist was very positive about the state of Huntington's disease research and clinical trials. He presented a future where an effective treatment for HD may only be another five or ten years away. I was a bit shocked by that. At the time, so shortly after my initial diagnosis, I was feeling like I'd been handed a death sentence and getting this information from him was a little ray of sunshine on a *very* cloudy day.

Neurologist

The Neurologist is most likely to be the healthcare professional whom will take the lead when it comes to managing your Huntington's disease; potentially for years to come, right through the in-between years and into the symptomatic years.

The Neurologist is the brain doctor and when it comes to Huntington's disease, looking after the brain is an important job.

During the in-between years, you may only see the Neurologist on a yearly basis or every six months, but it may be more frequently if you become involved with research in one way or another.

At these annual visits, the Neurologist will check you over, running you through some neurological tests to determine if you may or may not be demonstrating some HD related symptoms. For me, as an in-betweener, these neurological exams and their outcome are what I'm most interested in learning.

Or, most scared of.

I want to know if there is *any* sign at all that I may be starting to show symptoms.

I'm also a bit of a "symptom seeker." What I mean by that is, I tend to look at every single stumble and every forgotten name and immediately conclude that it's the result of Huntington's disease. Symptom seeking receives its own chapter in this book.

Reviewing these episodes and concerns with the Neurologist during my regular visits allows him to provide me with some reassurance that I'm not demonstrating any symptoms. It gives him the opportunity to tell me to calm the hell down.

Obtaining Neurologist care can be a struggle for people in more remote geographical areas. Personally, I have about a 1.5-hour drive to reach my Neurologist's office. I'm happy to make that trip however because I feel like I'm seeing one of the best Neurologists in the country. In my opinion, 1.5-hours is *close* if it gets you to one of the best.

1.5-hours can be insurmountable, however, if transportation is an issue.

There are countless Huntington's disease individuals and families across the world who are nowhere near a Neurologist office. What do they do? How do they get access to quality care? It can be a real problem.

Technology can help in some cases. For HD patients in remote areas, seeing their Neurologist for a routine visit can be done through a screen.

Video teleconferencing has become a common and beneficial way for patients to interact with their healthcare team. A Neurologist can gain a surprising amount of insight using these methods. Who knows where the future will take us as technology advances further?

I'm hoping for teleporters, personally.

Some Neurologists will also take trips to more remote areas to see Huntington's disease families.

Neurologists play a large part in the development and implementation of clinical studies and, of course, once our in-between years are done, the Neurologist plays a key role in symptom management and caregiver support.

Psychiatrist

A Psychiatrist is a healthcare professional that you may, or may not, see during your travel through the in-between years. They are the mental health expert who can prescribe medications and treat conditions such as depression, anxiety or irritability.

As everybody's experience with Huntington's disease is different, some people won't require this type of assistance while others may need help with optimizing mental health throughout the entire journey.

I have been to see a Psychiatrist and continue to do so regularly. I've had issues with anxiety for several years, and I also struggle with irritability and outbursts of anger.

Whether these symptoms have anything to do with HD or they're just the way I've developed as a person, who knows. I do take some medication, however, to help me keep them under control.

Counsellor

Counselling can be an essential component of our healthcare plan. It can help us work towards an overall sense of well-being by addressing psycho-social issues that affect us, our loved ones and our caregivers.

Counsellors can be Social Workers, Psychologists or some other professional trained to help identify concerns and work towards resolutions for both in-betweeners and loved ones.

Sometimes it can be difficult to let someone into our most private thoughts and concerns, but it's important to make our loved ones aware of these feelings. And they, in turn, make us aware of theirs.

The benefits of professional counselling can't be overstated.

Research team

Part of the Neurologist's team could be professionals, such as Nurses and Research Assistants, who are on staff to help with running research and clinical studies programs.

As an example, at my Neurologist's clinic, they have several staff members there to assist in Huntington's disease-related clinical studies and projects like Enroll-HD, to name just one.

Clinical studies and research will be discussed in the next chapter, so remember the name "Enroll-HD" as it will be making a return.

Chapter 7
Participating in Research

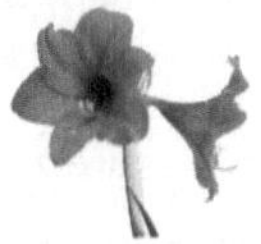

H untington's disease is a rare disease. The Huntington's disease Society of America presents this statistic on their website:

"Today, there are approximately 30,000 symptomatic Americans and more than 200,000 at-risk of inheriting the disease."

"30,000 symptomatic Americans." Although that sounds like a large number, in the big scheme of things, It's not.

Lisa Genova helps us give it some context in her book, *Inside the O'Briens*.

She suggests that if you took *all* the symptomatic HD individuals in the *whole* United States of America and put them in Boston's Fenway Park, they would fit comfortably. In fact, there would be more than 7,000 seats sitting empty.

30,000 is not a lot considering the population of the USA is about 325 million. Even when you throw in the 200,000 individuals estimated to be at risk for HD, it's still a drop in the bucket.

This example helps to demonstrate why participating in Huntington's disease research is so important. Good solid scientific evidence-based knowledge needs numbers to progress as quickly as possible.

It needs people. Both symptomatic individuals as well as the in-betweeners like us. It requires control subjects, like our gene-negative family members and loved ones. That's the key to rapidly progressing these clinical studies.

I'm all about speed here as I'm sure you are too.

With that said, it's not just about speed, but also quality. Science needs the right person for the right study and finding the right people for a study can be a significant portion of the work.

That's where programs like Enroll-HD can shine.

What is Enroll-HD?

Enroll-HD is an observational study. This means that it collects data from a person and then repeats that data collection at pre-determined intervals of time to learn how things change.

In Enroll-HD's case, the data is collected on a yearly basis. Here's more from the Enroll-HD website:

"Enroll-HD is a worldwide observational study for Huntington's disease families. It will monitor how the disease appears and changes over time in different people, and is open to people who either have HD or are at-risk. Enroll-HD is or will soon be up and running for HD families in North America, Europe, Latin America, Australia, New Zealand and some countries in Asia. It will eventually include more than 20,000 people. Monitoring people over time in a real-world setting contributes to scientific knowledge. The study is designed to accelerate the discovery and development of new therapeutics for HD."

Look at that number again:

"It will eventually include more than 20,000 people."

That's such a large number for one observational study when, again, you recall just how rare Huntington's disease is. Not only that, but this is a *worldwide* project. Look at the following map which demonstrates all the nations in the world where Enroll-HD is currently underway, or the plans are in the works:

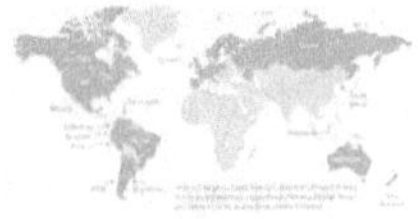

(Image: 8)

On the above map, countries in green are where Enroll-HD is currently underway or will soon begin, and the orange nations are candidates to join later.

Now *that* is an excellent pool of rich data that will only continue to grow and mature.

As I mentioned above, finding the right people for the right studies can be a very time-consuming task. This is another way that Enroll-HD is filling a critical role in the advancement of Huntington's disease clinical research.

Researchers can be granted access to the Enroll-HD database and use that treasure trove of information to search for appropriate people to act as subjects in their study. It's a huge time saver. The value of that time savings cannot be overstated as it relates to advancing these studies and working towards effective Huntington's disease treatments.

Getting involved in Enroll-HD

As an in-betweener, you are in no way obligated to participate in Enroll-HD or any other study for that matter. As I've said in previous chapters, you are 100% in charge of how you spend *your* in-between years.

If you do decide to go ahead and participate, it's entirely possible that your Neurologist is already involved with Enroll-HD. If not, they would be able to direct you to a clinic who is.

How to learn about other research opportunities

Many studies today recruit their subjects directly out of Enroll-HD, so if you are interested in becoming involved in Huntington's disease studies in general, start with getting yourself into the Enroll-HD database.

Once in there, you may start getting considered for studies before you know it.

I've been in the Enroll-HD program for two years and, during that time, I've been recruited into two studies and considered for a third.

Talk to your Neurologist, make sure they know you're interested, and do a little research yourself. Learn which studies are going on and where they are located. Huntington's disease Association websites will have information about trials and studies that are active or in the pipeline, so those sites are a great place to start.

Keeping up to date on research outcomes

Keeping up to date on Huntington's disease research news can be great, but also heartbreaking.

The news is great when we hear about advancements in a study or, we hear about all the exciting research that is in the planning stages. The news is heartbreaking when we hear about failures. So heartbreaking.

It's important to remember, scientists, learn a great deal from failures. In fact, some would say that it's the failures that advance the science! It's the failures that add to our body of knowledge on HD and move us a tad closer to a treatment. We need to learn about what doesn't work, so we know where to shift our focus.

The most trusted source for updates on Huntington's disease news and research is HDBuzz.net.

Full stop.

HDBuzz is run by Dr. Ed Wild and Dr. Jeff Carroll. They present the information in an honest and up-front manner and will let you know when a piece of HD news is something to be excited about, and when it's not.

Chapter 8
Symptom Seeking

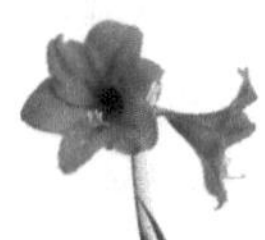

As an in-betweener, I've spent a great deal of my time "symptom seeking." I've mentioned this term in a previous chapter but let me remind you.

Symptom seeking is looking at every little stumble and every forgotten name and jumping to the conclusion that:

"Ah, it must be the HD!"

Of course, it's very likely *not* the HD, but it's hard not to have those thoughts.

Here's a perfect example:

Over the past year, I've had two falls. Both involved me tripping on something and going right down to the floor.

"No worries, right? Happens to everyone, right?"

"No, darn right it's a worry, it's the HD. THE H.D.!"

Each time (after some freaking out) I made a note of the falls and planned to bring them up on my next visit to the Neurologist. Once there, he proceeded to go through his regular neurological assessment and watch me do some walking and balance activities.

When I told him about the two falls, he didn't seem too concerned. He made notes about them, but not too concerned.

He said, and I'm paraphrasing here:

"Part of my job here is to look for any signs that may be the result of Huntington's disease symptoms and I don't see anything today that leads me to believe you have symptoms."

And, sigh.

(Of course, between you and me, I still think those falls were related to my HD. Or maybe they're not).

The example above was just one. I could list several others. What the heck, here's a list just off the top of my head:

- forgetting names

- mixing up toothbrushes

- fidgeting

- anytime I drop an object

- getting behind with work

- getting angry about something

- making a wrong turn while driving

I have blamed all those occurrences on Huntington's disease at some point or another, so you can see, I'm clearly a symptom seeker.

Perhaps as an in-betweener, you are as well.

And you know what? **It's 100% okay and normal**.

The benefit of predictive genetic testing is you know what's coming. That's also the problem with predictive genetic testing: *you know what's coming*!

You know, based on your CAG score, that it's likely to come at a certain point in your life and it's tough not always to have that in the back of your head.

> "Hello, it's me, your little gene mutation. I'm back here!"

Especially once you reach that "average age of onset" period in your life. Or, you reach the same age that your HD parent was when *they* started demonstrating symptoms.

It can feel like a ticking-time-bomb at that point.

The truth of the matter is that once we *do* start demonstrating symptoms, *we* probably won't be the ones noticing. It'll be our loved ones and family members. Those people in our lives who know us best, are likely to see any changes well before us in-betweeners.

In fact, lacking insight into your early symptom progression has been documented as being common in HD.

This from Bates, Tabrizi and Jones, (2014):

> "From the prodromal phase onward, impairment of insight into symptoms is a feature of HD. Indeed, it is

> axiomatic that a patient who is concerned about onset
> has probably not yet encountered it since the emer-
> gence of symptoms and signs is so often associated
> with a lack of awareness that it has occurred1."

"Prodromal phase" refers to the period in Huntington's disease where early symptoms are beginning to develop. Later in the book is a chapter devoted to the development of symptoms and we will revisit the prodromal phase then.

So, there you go. If we're insightful enough to notice that we forget people's names more often, it's probably got nothing to do with HD and has more to do with turning forty.

And getting gray hair. Which, may or may not, describe me perfectly.

So, what do we do about it?

The first thing is to understand that it is completely normal to symptom seek during these in-between years. We all do it from time-to-time. It's nothing to feel silly or guilty about.

Talking about your concerns can be exceedingly helpful. Having another in-betweener to run things by, either at a Chapter meeting or through online messaging or social media, will quickly demonstrate to you that you are not alone in this.

Raising your concerns with your Neurologist can be very helpful. Even if it's not your regular time for a check-up, give him or her a call. Chatting with an expert will no doubt help to ease the anxiety you're feeling.

And finally, as I've said before, *knowledge is power*. Learning more about the beast that ails you, including all the advancements that are taking place related to science's understanding of the disease, is key to easing the fear of the unknown.

Chapter 9

Fear

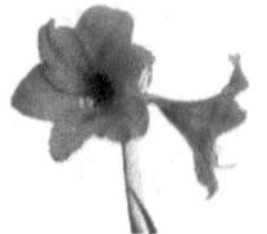

I'm scared.

I'm not going to lie. I am terrified. You can call me a "scaredy-pants" if you want to, I don't mind.

I've got several fears. Perhaps, as a fellow in-betweener, you have some too.

Or, maybe you don't, that can be a healthy mindset as well. As I've said before, everyone manages, and is in control, of their own in-between years, and there's no right or wrong way to *feel*.

Me, I'm scared.

I have many fears that mingle around in the back of my head, occasionally coming to the forefront when least expected. Usually when I'm at work and my mind wanders away from the task at hand, or in the evening when I'm playing with my kids.

Each person likely has their own unique set of fears. Everyone's life experience is different.

- maybe you have kids; maybe you don't

- maybe you're young; maybe you're older

- maybe you're new to HD; maybe you've cared for numerous family members

This chapter is going to be very personal, full of my fears and worries. It's not my wish to be so gloomy and negative, but I want you to know that you are not alone if you share similar concerns.

Fear of being a burden

I'm married with two young kids. My extended family lives hours away by car, so there's no doubt that my wife will be handling my care when it's needed, mostly on her own.

I worry about how that will affect her. The way this disease usually strikes people in their prime is so tragic.

And remember, the *caregiver* is in their prime *too*.

It's *so* tragic.

I know that if you were to ask my wife, she would immediately tell you that she is not concerned about her potential caregiver role. She would say something along the lines of:

"I married him in sickness and health."

But still, I hate that she might have to go through that in her young future.

Fear of not being there for my kids

This is probably my biggest fear, and it's the one that upsets me the most and keeps me up at night.

Now that I'm a father, I've realized the joy of watching my kids experience and learn new things. Even seemingly small achievements, like becoming competent at zipping a coat, turns me into a mushy mess of proud-daddiness.

I don't want to lose that.

I don't want *them* to lose that father figure in their life.

I want to be around to talk to my boy about baseball and girls. I want to be a good male role model for my daughter, so she can learn what a good man is.

Even as I write this, I'm tearing up; it affects me so much.

Fear that my kids may have inherited the HD gene from me

I think all parents with kids at risk for inheriting the Huntington's disease gene likely have this fear. Maybe mixed with a serving of guilt.

It wasn't until about a year after my youngest child was born that I began to think I may be at risk for HD. Prior to that, in my mind, I was in the clear.

In retrospect, I should have thought about it, but it *never* entered my mind.

Now that I know I'm positive, I've spent a lot of time thinking about our family planning and wondering *why* it never came up with our prenatal healthcare practitioners.

I remember sitting in the exam room with my wife as we went through the initial appointment with the midwife. I remember her asking both my wife and myself about our medical histories.

Did I mention Huntington's disease?

I know I mentioned the Spina Bifida on my mom's side of the family, *but did I bring up the HD*?

I don't remember. If I did, I would think the midwife would dig a bit deeper into the possibility of me undergoing genetic testing, just to be safe. But, maybe I felt so safe about my risk that it never even occurred to me to bring it up. Perhaps Huntington's disease is so rare, that she never thought to ask more about it.

That's where my feelings of guilt stem from.

If I had thought I was at risk, I would have undergone the predictive testing and done things a bit differently, but I can't change the past. I have two kids whom I love more than *anything in the world,* and there's no way around the fact that Huntington's disease is going to be a big part of their lives moving forward.

Fear of the unknown

One of the nasty things about Huntington's disease, and these in-between years in particular, is just not knowing what is in store for us.

Sure, our CAG score can give us an idea of when symptoms might begin for us, but we don't know what those symptoms may look like.

Everyone with Huntington's disease presents a little bit differently, and I've seen HD symptomatic folks continue to work and keep hold of their cognition well into the disease progression.

On the other hand, I've seen people lose their personality and lose their grip on reality quite early on.

This terrifies me.

How will *my* mind keep it together?

I feel that I can handle the chorea and even the mood swings; I mean, there are medications that can help control or minimize those symptoms, right?

But losing my grip on reality, and not knowing when it may happen, is a huge fear of mine.

Fear that there won't be an effective treatment for my kids if they need it

When my mom and dad had kids back in the early seventies, it was already understood that my grandmother likely had Huntington's disease, although there was no testing process in those days.

The doctors told my parents that they should not have children to reduce the risk of spreading the mutation further.

They made the complex decision of moving ahead with building a family and decided to keep it to two children, rather than have the larger family that my mother wanted back in those days. (I previously mentioned that I have a younger sister who tested negative for Huntington's disease. She is a half-sister from my dad's second marriage which is why I'm not mentioning her here.)

My mom has told me that she was convinced, back in the seventies, that scientists would develop some treatment or cure by the time either my sister or I may need it as adults.

Thirty or forty years in the future sounds like a long time, and it is really. Here we are, forty years on, and still no effective treatment or cure.

I mention this story because I think of it every time I have the exact same thought about my kids:

"Ah, they're so close to a treatment now. I have no doubt there will be something for my kids when they grow up if they need it."

I've said that many times.

My mom said the same thing forty years ago. What if there isn't *something*?

Fear that there won't be an effective treatment for me before I'm lost

I mentioned in the chapter I wrote about different healthcare professionals you may meet, that the Geneticist told me something following my predictive testing that I needed to hear.

He said to me that an effective treatment for Huntington's disease might be only five or ten years away. He described all the positive and exciting research that is in the pipeline, including some that may be ready in time for me to benefit from.

I was *blown* away by that.

As I mentioned before, initially following my positive test, I was convinced that my life was close to being done and over with, so this was very good to hear.

But what if it's not ready for me? What if I'm well into my symptomatic phase of the disease long before something comes along and it's too late?

This crosses my mind every time I open an article or read a study related to Huntington's disease.

"Oh, please let this be good news!"

I say with my fingers crossed as I begin to read.

Chapter 10
When Do I Tell People About My Huntington's Disease?

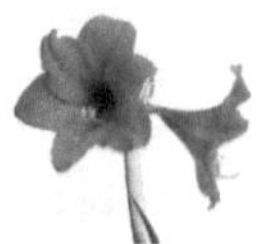

The decision to tell someone about your Huntington's disease is an extremely personal one. Almost as personal as the decision to be tested in the first place. This fact can be even more apparent during the in-between years when you could be decades away from any signs of the disease or decline in your health.

It's entirely possible that you decide to tell *nobody* outside of your immediate family if even them.

That's okay. As I said, it's an incredibly *personal* decision that is *yours* to make.

Yours.

It could be that you value privacy and would just rather not share your HD diagnosis with any more people than completely necessary.

Me? I shared my diagnosis on *Facebook*. With everyone.

Here's the post from July 12, 2015:

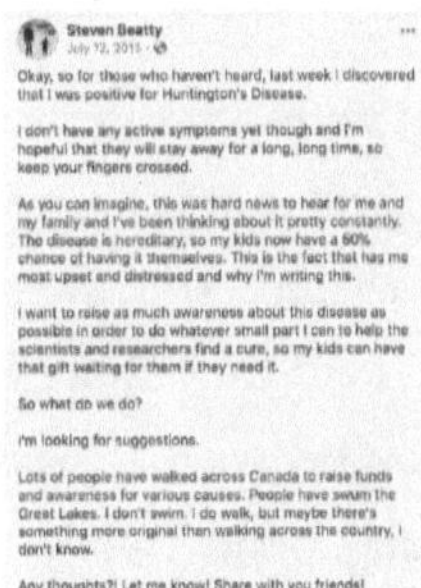

(Image: https://facebook.com/stevenbeatty)

Yup, shared with everyone. And no, I haven't walked across Canada. Yet.

My point is (and you'll see this is a recurring theme in this series), everyone assesses their situation through their own lens. People are completely free to act in whatever way they choose.

If you want to tell the world? That's fine.

If you choose to keep your HD a secret, that's fine as well.

There are likely numerous factors that may influence your decision about sharing your diagnosis versus keeping it secret. Genetic and workplace discrimination may be one. Obtaining health and life insurance may be another.

Countless factors. Too many to be addressed in one chapter if it was even possible to identify them all.

The following pages touch on some of the more common issues and are intended to help facilitate your own thinking and reflection on what's essential for *you*.

Ultimately, it's always recommended to speak with a genetic counsellor about these concerns as the results of undergoing predictive testing and sharing the results can have implications reaching far and wide.

That's what the genetic counsellors are there for and why it's often a prerequisite before clinics will even test you for Huntington's disease.

Also, the scope of this chapter is not to provide legal advice, and it should not be considered so. If you require specific legal information about something that you believe may be discrimination based on your HD predictive testing, please contact a legal office for proper guidance.

Work

Many in-betweeners will decide not to share their Huntington's disease diagnosis with their places of employment. There's no need to if you're happily working away and are exhibiting no signs of the disease that may be interfering with your work or jeopardizing the safety of you or a third party.

You have every right to keep your HD a secret. And, you have every right to tell your employer if that's what you decide you want to do.

Your situation will influence your decision significantly.

If you're a young in-betweener, just starting your career with hopes of climbing that corporate ladder, you may be more apt to keep your HD to yourself. If you are in your forties, comfortable with where you are in life and with all your insurance and healthcare benefits set up and ready to go, then you may be more comfortable sharing.

Regardless of what choices you make, there are laws in most developed countries that prevent an employer from discriminating against someone in the workplace based on their positive HD testing. Doing so would be considered genetic discrimination.

Genetic Discrimination

Genetic discrimination is defined as occurring:

"When people are treated differently by their employer or insurance company because they have a gene mutation that causes or increases the risk of an inherited disorder."

As I mentioned previously, most countries have laws in place to make this discrimination illegal, and for good reasons. Insurance companies would no doubt raise your premiums if they knew you were likely to develop some debilitating condition later in life. These laws prevent them from using or requiring genetic information when deciding on a person's insurance coverage.

Below are two examples of laws in place to prevent this type of discrimination.

Genetic Information Non-Discrimination Act (GINA)

In the United States, there is a federal law called the Genetic Information Non-Discrimination Act (GINA). Not only does GINA prevent insurance companies from using your predictive genetic testing against you, but it also:

"Makes it illegal for employers to use a person's genetic information when making decisions about hiring, promotion, and several other terms of employment9."

Genetic Non-Discrimination Act (GNA)

Canada has been lagging when it comes to putting anti-genetic discrimination laws into place. Only as of 2017 has the Genetic Non-Discrimination Act (GNA) been made law, but there continues to be a debate about what the final law will look like, and it's not a completely done deal as of the time this book was published5.

Family and Friends

I learned very quickly, once I entered the in-between years, that there was no greater source of support than my family and friends.

They are my foundation.

They knock sense into me when I'm blabbering on about how I have noticed 27 new Huntington's disease-related symptoms in myself.

They will be there in the future to hold me up, keep me safe and make my decisions when I'm no longer able to.

Again, who you choose to share your HD diagnosis with is one hundred percent your choice. If there's one thing that I can say, it's this: having a loved one (family or friend) with whom you can talk about your feelings and thoughts and fears, can be so significant. Especially, when it comes to maintaining a positive and healthy mindset as you move through these in-between years.

We've all heard the phrase:

"Don't keep things all bottled up inside. It's not healthy!"

There's a lot of truth to that old cliché!

Dating

Dating during the in-between years can be, without question, a complicated and often stressful undertaking.

Determining the *right* time to tell a potential romantic partner about your Huntington's disease can be difficult.

Should you tell them on the first date?

Should you wait until the feelings are stronger?

The best answer to these questions is likely this: not too soon and not too late. How's that for vague?

Revealing your in-betweener status to a potential partner on the first date or so, may instantly build a wall between the two of you getting to know each other at all. They may decide not to move forward with getting to know more about you because they've run head-on into this wall and that will put an end to it.

Yes, you will need to tell them. But, give it some time. Learn about each other.

I read somewhere that, yes, Huntington's disease is a big part of our in-betweener life, but it's *one* part of who we are.

That's important to remember.

Sure, you have HD. But you're also a painter. You like to surf. Your dream is to travel to Nepal. Your favourite colour is blue. You can breakdance. You speak Spanish.

There is so *much* about *you*, that is *more* than the HD.

Let any potential mate see and learn all those awesome things about you. As you learn more about them.

There are no rules about dating during these in-between years. You'll likely know when it's the right time to share your Huntington's disease when the moment arrives.

Children

Introducing your Huntington's disease status to your children is another experience that many in-betweeners are dreading; myself included.

For children, learning about HD in the family will be undoubtedly overwhelming, for so many reasons. The information given to them, and when, will of course depend on the age of the child.

Perhaps as an in-betweener, you can remember yourself being told about your family's Huntington's disease history. Were you a teenager? Younger?

Drawing upon that experience may be helpful as you plan to introduce the HD to *your* children.

Keeping the information age appropriate is vital. This following quote is taken from the Huntington's Disease Society of America's resource booklet entitled "Talking with Kids":

"Giving your child information about HD – the right amount at the right age – will give him or her tools to deal with the changes in the family while helping him or her to feel secure and live positively."

This above-mentioned resource is one of many fantastic sources of information available for us in-betweeners. Many can be found on your Association's website and are written by some brilliant professionals trained in complex areas, like introducing Huntington's disease to children.

Chapter 11
Anger

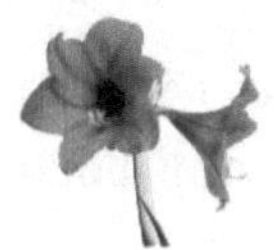

When it comes to Huntington's disease, there are a lot of things to be angry about. I certainly am.

- I'm angry that I tested positive.

- I'm angry that my kids are now at risk.

- I'm angry that I might miss out on so much of life.

- I'm angry that I might not get to enjoy a retirement.

- I'm angry because I feel like I'm being ripped off.

I could go on and on.

Why Do We Feel Anger?

Often, anger is a symptom of something else, like frustration. Perhaps fear. Perhaps sadness. Maybe even emerging psychological symptoms related to the Huntington's disease.

Whatever the cause may be, the anger can explode to the surface very quickly.

When the anger does surface, it tends to explode all over the people we love most: our spouses, our kids.

I get angry from frustration or being overwhelmed. There have been many times that my wife has taken the brunt of that from me. In fact, I'm convinced she's a saint, but that's a story for another day.

What Do We Do About It?

Years ago, I read a sign somewhere that had this statement on it:

"Anger is one letter away from danger."

Cheesy, yes. But, that little seven-word sentence has stayed with me for years, and I think of it often.

I try to think of it when the anger is controlling me. I know that nothing good is going to come from heading down that road to danger.

As I mentioned at the beginning of this chapter, there's a great deal for us in-betweeners to be angry about. There's no question about that.

That doesn't mean we should curl up into an angry ball and do nothing. We must fight the anger. We must figure out what is triggering the anger. Search for that cause. Have open conversations about it with our loved ones and our healthcare team.

Counselling can be a huge help here, specifically when it comes to developing strategies that you can put into place when you sense that anger beginning to bubble.

Medications can go a long way in many cases, for example, if you struggle with anxiety or depression. Don't be shy about bringing it up with the doctor, even if they don't ask. Write down your concerns on a sheet of paper, so you don't forget to mention it the next time you're there. Be honest about it. That's the key to finding solutions.

You'll never be able to erase the emotion of anger from your life altogether, but by developing strategies to minimize it, you can help to reduce the number of trips you take down that road to (d)anger.

Chapter 12
Making Babies

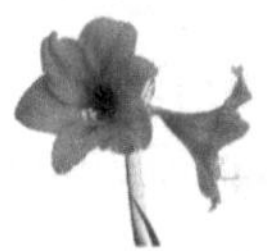

The desire to produce offspring is human nature. It's part of what being a living creature is all about. Finding a mate, joining together and mixing genes to create a beautiful bouncing baby girl or boy is at the core of our being.

Oh right, *genes*.

As an in-betweener, there isn't much that's more frightening than thinking about passing genes on to the next generation. Well, one particular gene anyway.

Back in chapter three of this book, while discussing what Huntington's disease is, I touched on the fact that HD is an autosomal dominant disorder. Let's refresh our memories. An autosomal dominant disorder is a:

"Pattern of inheritance in which an affected individual has one copy of a mutant gene and one normal gene on a pair of autosomal chromosomes. Individuals with autosomal dominant diseases have a

50/50 chance of passing the mutant gene and therefore the disorder on to each of their children."

That pesky Huntington's disease gene mutation within all of us in-betweeners means that each of our kids will have a 50% chance of inheriting our bad copy.

Not good.

Countless HD couples have struggled with this knowledge over the years and decades. Their conversations no doubt including the following questions:

- "Is it even fair to bring a kid into this world knowing they have a 50/50 chance of inheriting this damn disease?"

- "If we don't have kids at all, then we can stop this line of the disease right here. It would stop with me, right?"

I'm reminded of the first sentence of this chapter: *The desire to produce offspring is human nature*. Is a person, a *couple*, to be denied that right just because of the Huntington's disease?

No, they're not. *We're* not.

There are options available today for HD couples looking to start a family. Your access to these options may depend on where you are in the world and, in some cases, what you can afford or have covered through health insurance, but there is some choice here.

Sperm or Egg Donation

Using a sperm or egg donor is an option for some couples. This process is completed through a donation clinic with qualified donors.

A donated egg or sperm is used in place of the partner who has the Huntington's disease gene mutation, thus ensuring that no HD related genetics make it to the baby. The donated egg or sperm is combined with the non-HD partner's egg or sperm in the lab and then implanted into the uterus of our female.

As I mentioned, there are no HD related genes passed on in this method which ensures that the baby will not grow up to develop Huntington's disease. This fact also means; however, that the HD member of this parenting team will not be considered the biological parent of the child.

Access to, and affordability of, this procedure will vary depending on where you are in the world. As with so many of these options.

Prenatal Diagnosis (PD)

Prenatal diagnosis is an option for HD parents and involves testing the fetus in utero for the Huntington's disease gene mutation. This testing occurs in early pregnancy (at about 10–15 weeks depending on the method used by the physician) to obtain the fetus' DNA.

If the testing comes back as positive for the HD mutation, then it would mean that the fetus will develop Huntington's disease later in life and the pregnancy would be terminated. If there is no mutation seen in the testing, then the child will grow up to be HD free.

For couples deciding to use prenatal testing as an option, they:

"Need to be counselled beforehand about PD only being an appropriate option if they would choose to terminate an affected fetus. This would otherwise lead to the highly undesirable situation of parents knowing about a child's mutation-positive result from birth1."

This fact is important to remember. The decision to have an abortion if the fetus comes back as positive for HD needs to be discussed by both future mom and future dad. Be sure to talk about this a great deal beforehand and don't be afraid to access the advice of a genetic counsellor.

Preimplantation Genetic Diagnosis (PGD) In-Vetro Fertilization (IVF)

Preimplantation Genetic Diagnosis (PGD) is another process completed in a laboratory. The potential parents, both the HD affected, and non-HD affected, provide samples of their eggs and sperm which are then fertilized.

Once embryos are formed, they are tested for the HD gene mutation. The positive embryos are disposed of, and the ones that are negative for HD are implanted in the uterus through in-vetro fertilization (IVF).

The success rate for this procedure can vary, but the literature seems to point to around 1 in 3.

As the embryos implanted into the womb do not have the Huntington's disease gene mutation, they will not grow up to develop HD later in life.

Non-Disclosure or Exclusion Testing

The techniques discussed above are great options for couples who know the Huntington's disease status of the partner at risk. But, what if the partner at risk has *not* undergone HD predictive testing *and* did not want to.

For that, there is an option called Non-Disclosure or Exclusion Testing. This process requires another member of the family to be involved: the HD at-risk partner's HD affected parent. Wow, that's confusing.

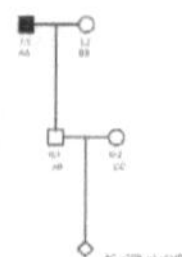

Refer to the chart above and let's assume you are a person at risk for inheriting Huntington's disease from your father, but you haven't been tested yet. In the chart above, you would be the white square "AB." Your father, who we know has HD is the black square "AA." That's your mom over there at "BB" and your spouse next to you there at "CC."

Your future baby is the diamond at the bottom.

Blood samples are collected from you, your father and the embryo. The scientists look for markers related to the section of the DNA where the Huntington disease gene mutation may be. It's possible to see whether the fetus seems to have inherited that section from your affected father.

Argh, my brain is hurting!

If the fetus has not inherited that section from your father, then the chances of the baby inheriting HD is very low.

If the fetus has inherited that section from your father, then the chances of the baby inheriting HD is 50%.

Exclusion testing can be completed for a fetus in-utero, like the prenatal diagnosis, as well as in a petri dish, similar to the Preimplantation Genetic Diagnosis with IVF.

Ugh, I need a nap. Oh wait, there's more!

Natural

If none of these medically assisted procedures are affordable or accessible to you, or they don't appeal to you and your partner, you can, of course, continue with having children the old-fashioned natural way.

These are *your* choices as a couple to make. Again, how you manage *your* in-between years is up to you. And your partner in this case. Talking to a genetic counsellor about your choice to proceed with a natural pregnancy will ensure you are moving forward with a decision that's well informed.

Having a child naturally will result in each child having a 50% chance of inheriting the Huntington gene.

Adoption

Adoption is an option for in-betweeners to consider as well. The process for this will vary from place to place, and again your local genetic counsellor or Huntington's disease Association can provide you with information.

Chapter 13
Staying Positive

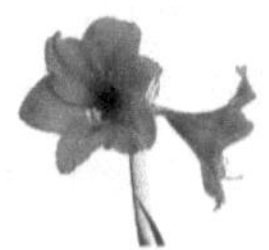

Maintaining a positive attitude can be a daunting task while facing a future with Huntington's disease. Daunting, not only for us in-betweeners, but also for our families and loved ones.

How do we stay positive?

I'll be honest, for me, there have been days where I've felt down in the dumps. I've had days where I've said to myself something like this:

> "To hell with it. What's the point? I'll just quit my job, start smoking again and sit on the porch all day. Why not do that?"

I haven't followed through on those negative thoughts, well at least not so far, but it's hard not to think that way occasionally.

So, where can we find support?

Family and Friends

Our family and friends are often our strongest and most loyal source of support. They know us when we are at our lowest, our highest and everything in between.

Most times, in the company of our family and friends, we have no social barriers up masking how we're feeling. They can see what's going on and will want to be there for us.

We feel accountable to them and don't want to let them down. Often, that can be enough to keep us off the porch.

Don't hesitate to reach out to them. Chances are, if you're not feeling yourself or are going through a particularly negative period, they'll already know it. Like I said, no one knows you better than your family and friends.

Support from Other In-Betweeners

Following my Huntington's disease predictive testing I started becoming involved with the Huntington Society. As I mentioned back in chapter 5, being more involved with my local Huntington's disease Association was a huge benefit for me, for many reasons.

One key reason, however, was meeting other in-betweeners like myself. Like you.

Huntington's disease is no longer a disease that's in the shadows. It's no longer a disease that families hide away in upstairs bedrooms and long-term care facilities.

Now that genetic discrimination laws are on the books in many places, HD families and in-betweeners have less fear being open about their genetic mutation. They are more likely to get out there and become active in fundraising and community events.

The very first Huntington Society of Canada event that my wife and I went to was an education presentation, mainly focused on what was new in HD research. At that event, we met a family that we've been connected to ever since.

In fact, one part of that family is a mirror image of my wife and me; it's freaky.

- they're a married couple like us

- they have two young kids, almost the same age as ours

- they live; literally, a five-minute drive from us and our kids now go to the same school

- he lives at risk for HD

My long-winded point is, they have become our friends, and I have no doubt that as the years go by, they will end up being an essential support for us. And I hope, us for them if they need it.

We likely never would have met and realized our HD connection without the Association.

Counselling

Counselling can be beneficial if you're having issues maintaining positivity.

I know, I know. Yuck, Counselling.

It can be hard to open yourself up to someone in the way a counsellor is skilled at encouraging, but it can be so beneficial to you if you allow it.

I've been to a counsellor, a couple of years before I knew about my Huntington's disease. My long-standing issues with anxiety took me there, and I found it quite helpful.

The counsellor raised the possibility of me going on an anti-anxiety medication. She arranged an appointment for me with a physician to be assessed for that possibility. Initiating that course of treatment for my anxiety proved to be hugely beneficial for me, and I'm not sure that I would have come to that conclusion on my own without the help of a counsellor.

Now, I'm not saying medication is the cure-all for everything. Not at all. In fact, often a counsellor can help us get to the bottom of our emotional issues without pharmacological interventions. But, in my example, I turned out to benefit from both courses of treatment.

Medications

Some physicians will prescribe medication for everything, and some will be more reluctant.

My philosophy is this: if your emotional or psychological concern can be managed *without* medication, then that's all the better.

Today's medications tend to be quite safe and well researched, but if they can be avoided, then why not avoid them?

With that said, I do take medication for anxiety, as I mentioned previously, and I find it very helpful. I didn't hesitate to try it, and my doctor is there to monitor it as needed.

If your difficulty maintaining positivity during these in-between years is the result of clinical depression or something along those lines, then being treated with appropriate medication can be life-changing.

Talk to your doctor. Add it to that list of questions that you are bringing to your next appointment. Go ahead, write it down. Right now.

Exercise, and More Exercise

When it comes to maintaining a positive attitude, there may be nothing as important to us in-betweeners then exercise.

Exercise is so important that the next chapter will be dedicated solely to it, so keep yourself on the edge of your seat.

Or, go for a run and then come back and read it.

Food for Positive Thought

Before leaving this chapter, here's a reminder: *There is so much to feel positive about today!*

I've heard people say comments like this: "There has never been a better time to have Huntington's disease than today!" I'm not a big fan of that statement, but I understand what point they are trying to get across.

Science is so close to an effective treatment to delay the onset of HD symptoms. It *will* happen. It's just a matter of time.

As you read this, clinical trials are happening with in-betweeners like us taking new compounds to learn their effects and safety. Not only that, but there are numerous other studies in the planning stages that are coming down that old pipeline.

Stay positive.

Soon you can toss this book in the garbage because there will be no need for it.

Chapter 14

Exercise

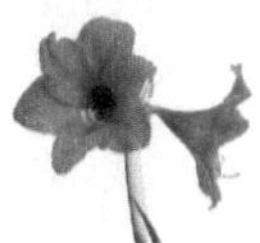

The importance of exercise for those of us in the in-between years cannot be exaggerated.

Over the years and decades, there have been many research studies completed with a focus on identifying *something* that will delay the onset of Huntington's disease symptoms.

Something. *Anything*.

Scientists have studied food. They've looked at various medicinal compounds. Different lifestyle factors have been investigated.

So far, the only factor that seems to show some promise in delaying symptom onset in HD is exercise.

I say "seems to show" because the scientific body of knowledge is still growing, but there may be a correlation here. A lifestyle consisting of regular exercise *may* delay the onset of Huntington's disease-related symptoms.

For me, "may delay onset" is good enough. Exercise is something everyone should be doing for improved overall health anyway, so if there's some added benefit for us in-betweeners, then all the better.

What is Exercise Anyway?

Exercise is more than just being active. Being active is great, don't get me wrong, but *exercise* gets the heart and lungs working. Here's a good description:

> "Exercise is a specific form of physical activity – planned, purposeful physical activity performed with the intention of acquiring fitness or other health benefits. Working out at a health club, swimming, cycling, running, and sports, like golf and tennis, are all forms of exercise."

Generally speaking, the conventional wisdom nowadays is to perform about 30 minutes of good aerobic exercise every day, such as running, swimming or going to the gym and weight training, that kind of thing.

Get that heart pumping and those lungs expanding!

Exercise is Good for Your Psychological Health

We all know that exercise is good for our physical health, but the benefits to our *psychological* health, or our overall sense of well-being, is paramount.

Being active and getting outside if you're able, can be fantastic for your spirit. It fills your body with Vitamin D and gets that well-oxygenated blood pumping strongly into every nook and cranny.

This fact has been hammered into me at almost every physician visit I've have had along my journey through the in-between years, from my Neurologist to my Psychiatrist.

Not everyone loves, or finds enjoyment, with the outdoors. Find what works for *you* and keep that spirit happy. It will go a long way in maintaining your quality of life as you move through the in-between years.

Exercise and Your Heart

There is some evidence in the literature that suggests Huntington's disease affects the heart in some way. It seems that it may have something to do with the conduction of the heart.

Heart failure is documented as being a cause of death in HD. The reasons are not clear, but this could be an excellent example of how Huntington's disease affects the body in areas other than the brain.

If you have been living a bit of a sedentary lifestyle without too much activity, speak with your physician before jumping head-on into a strenuous exercise routine.

Be a Good Role Model

If there's one thing I've learned since becoming a parent, it's this: Those kids are watching and hearing everything you do.

And I mean everything. If you drop the "f-word" during breakfast, the kids are repeating it during kindergarten share time.

Their brains are little sponges. Everything is being soaked up and filed away as they develop into little people. They are learning how to *be* people, and it's by watching us that they do this.

That not only goes for "f-words," but also for lifestyle decisions. They watch us to learn what a healthy way of living is. If they grow up seeing us exercise regularly, then they'll see that as being what's normal.

Why am I talking about role modelling? What does it have to do with the in-between years?

Our kids will look to us as an example for how someone copes with Huntington's disease. Not only HD but chronic illness in general, for that matter.

If they see us giving up and not doing all we can to make the best of what we've been given, then they'll take that message further into their lives. For those of us who have children at risk for Huntington's disease themselves, we need to show them what fighting looks like.

We need to show them that we did all we could to fight that cursed disease and did *not* give up. We need to show our kids what a true Huntington's disease warrior is.

That includes exercise. I'm sorry to break the news to your glutes.

Chapter 15

Caring

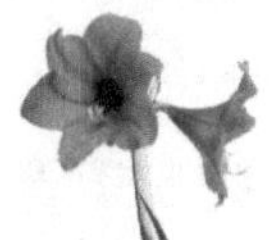

The heritability of Huntington's disease is a large part of what makes the disease so cruel and unkind. It indeed is a family disease, and for those of us from HD families, that fact is no more apparent than during the in-between years.

It's during that time that we may be directly faced with Huntington's disease on a multi-generational level.

- we might see it in an HD symptomatic parent

- we might be anticipating the future of our own Huntington's disease or caring for HD symptomatic siblings

- we might be fearing for the future of our children who may be at risk for HD

In all these cases, those of us in the in-between years may find ourselves involved in the role of *caregiver*. Along with other members of our families, a significant majority of our time may be devoted to this role.

As I've mentioned before, professionally, I work as a Registered Nurse in the home care sector. Every day I see caregivers caring for loved ones, and I observe first hand how challenging that role can be. I see caregivers burning out and, after years of looking after a spouse or a parent, are having to move that loved one to long-term care.

It's a heartbreaking journey these caregivers move through. Watching the deterioration of a spouse who once was so strong that he carried his new wife over the threshold of the house he built. Watching a mom who carried her kids around the house on her back.

Now, watching them move into long-term care.

It's so emotional for everyone involved.

For us in-betweeners, caring for Huntington's disease parents, we are involved in this heartbreaking journey, all the time wondering about our own HD future. Wondering how long until *our* heartbreaking journey begins.

Preventing Caregiver Burnout

Caregiver burnout is extremely common. If you're struggling with your role as a caregiver, do not feel that you are failing in any way. Do not judge yourself and wonder why other people can care for their loved one without any issues and you're not.

Everybody struggles. *Everybody* has that same internal dialogue about being a failure.

They are not, and you are not. Trust me. As I said, I see this every day.

The key to managing caregiver burnout is twofold. Firstly, as I mentioned, stop judging yourself and calling yourself a failure. Doing so will open you up to the second point which is accepting help. Permit yourself to obtain some respite or caregiver relief.

Caregiver burnout is so common that many nations in the world have some respite support services built into some government funding. It's not uncommon to see adult day programs (safe places for adults with a cognitive decline to go and participate in programs and experience social interaction) or respite services through home care (support workers coming into homes allowing caregivers to get out for some time) accessible in communities around the world.

Family support can also be paramount in preventing caregivers from experiencing burnout.

Following my positive Huntington's disease genetic test, I began meeting and interacting with other HD families. One fact that always stuck out to me was how often HD families share in the caring of their symptomatic members.

It really is a family disease.

If you are interested in learning more about what specific caregiver supports are available in your area, contact your Huntington's disease Association, such as the Huntington's Disease Society of America. The HDSA also has some excellent caregiver literature on its website available to all.

Seeing Our Future as we Care for HD Symptomatic Parents

As I mentioned previously, for those of us in the in-between years, we may look to our symptomatic parent and wonder:

- "Is this how I'm going to go?"

- "Are my kids going to have to watch me deteriorate like this?"

There's no doubt that these thoughts can be unpleasant. Being face-to-face with our mortality can be terrifying.

It can also be empowering.

Take the negative self-talk and energy and turn them around to be positive. Don't be controlled by this disease that hasn't burdened you with symptoms yet. Get outside and be active with whatever activity you find pleasure in. Paint. Swim. Mobile app development.

Whatever.

I've said it before, and I'll say it again. *You are so much more than just Huntington's disease.* Don't forget about all those other great pieces of you that make you, *you*.

Chapter 16
Guilt

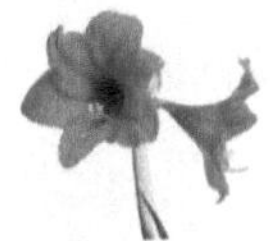

Following my Huntington's disease predictive testing positive result, my mother was quite distraught. I know that's probably stating the obvious. She was also expressing feelings of guilt. Guilt that she was somehow at fault in the whole scenario.

There's entirely no reason for her to feel this way, but there it was. On more than one occasion, she's even gone so far as to apologize to my sister and me for our HD diagnosis'.

I've asked her why she felt the need to apologize, and she had a difficult time answering. She seemed to be feeling guilty for having kids at risk for Huntington's disease in the first place. Like maybe she shouldn't have had kids at all.

Personally, I'm glad that I exist, and she is too. So, neither of us would want her to change anything if faced with the same decisions.

So, why the guilt?

The reality is, guilt may be one of many emotions felt by a parent upon the discovery that a child has inherited the Huntington's disease gene mutation from them. My mom was feeling guilty, and she wasn't even the parent with the HD gene.

Fear.

Sorrow.

Anger.

Name the emotion, and I'm sure it can be found in that psychological cocktail.

Within Huntington's disease families, we can see guilt experienced in numerous ways, which is why it has its own chapter in this book.

Not only can we see the parent guilt, as discussed above, but we can also see siblings experiencing a type of survivor's guilt if they test negative in their HD predictive testing.

Also, in-betweeners may experience guilt stemming from thoughts that they haven't done enough. That they haven't taken sufficient steps to plan for their kid's future or done enough to demonstrate to their spouse how much they mean to them.

What to Do About Guilt?

So, what do we do about all this guilt floating around like balloons at a birthday party?

Firstly, for the parent guilt related to passing along the Huntington's disease gene to the next generation. This form of guilt can be challenging to resolve, and for some people who experience it, it may never completely settle.

You need to communicate what you're feeling. Talk to your loved ones. Talk to a counsellor. Communication is the magic elixir for many things that ail us.

It's true.

Secondly, for the siblings experiencing survivor's guilt. It's quite a common experience, so don't feel guilty about feeling guilty! Again, communication is vital here. Talk about it with your brother or sister. And, let me tell you this: Learning that your HD result was negative, was one of the best things to ever happen to your HD positive sibling. They were elated and relieved on your behalf.

I can write until I'm blue in the face telling you that there's nothing to feel guilty about for possessing an unmutated HD gene, but I won't. I don't look good in blue. And, I have no right to tell you how to feel.

Be honest and reach out for support if you need it.

Finally, for those of us in the in-between years feeling that we have not done enough. Well, start doing things.

Sit down and make a list. Brainstorm some things that you can start doing to plan for the future.

You won't think of everything in one sitting. Keep an ongoing list in your phone or journal so you can add items to it as they pop into your head. A future chapter of this book will cover advanced planning, such as deciding on a Power of Attorney and insurance. These are tasks that you can begin to initiate now to help ease the guilt associated with concern that you are not doing enough.

Consider all those experiences that you want to provide for your spouse and your kids and other friends and loved ones. If you're feeling guilty about not doing enough, then start doing.

Chapter 17

Journaling

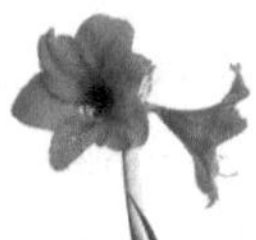

If there were a support group for journal addiction, I would be in it. There's not much that makes me happier than opening my favourite smartphone journaling app and filling it up with information on whatever is going on.

My journaling has evolved from consisting of the odd notation here and there to becoming a daily "lifelog" of my activities. It's filled with snapshots of my children, house renovations, and probably every date night that my wife and I have been on in the last four years.

In fact, let's look, so you know I'm authentic here. Here's a portion of a screenshot from the DayOne app on my iPhone.

(Image: Steven Beatty)

You can see that I have 7155 entries into this application over the past four years including 3759 photographs.

"Yes, my name is Steven Beatty, and I am a journaling addict."

Many people find journaling to be therapeutic. They find that writing their thoughts down onto paper, or into a computer, can be a great way to relieve tension and increase their understanding of why they are feeling a certain way.

When I began journaling, that was my initial plan, to record my thoughts on what was making me happy or sad or angry. But, my journaling has evolved into a recording of my daily activities and experiences.

Not only mine but my wife and kids as well.

Every day, I snap pictures and jot down notes on what's going on and what we are doing. If we've gone to the kid's hockey or soccer, I take a quick picture with a sentence or two of text and file it away.

I'm logging my life. I'm documenting my kid's lives through my eyes and, my thought is, it will be there for them to look at in the future if they so choose.

Smartphone Application

There are many journaling smartphone applications in all ecosystems, so if you use an iPhone or an Android phone, not to worry, there will be something there for you to use. I use DayOne on my iPhone, and it also has a Mac application that syncs very well with the desktop.

DayOne is beautiful, comfortable and it's a joy to use. As I mentioned above, I have thousands of entries in it.

- My son's birth.

- Our family vacations.

- My Huntington's disease predictive testing experience.

In fact, here's the entry immediately following my learning that my HD test came back positive:

Thu, Jul 9, 2015   •••

July 9, 2015 @ 1:44 PM

I just received a call from the genetics centre and it turns out I am positive for Huntington's Disease. I am extremely shocked and stunned. I have an appointment next week, on July 16, to go back to the genetics centre and get the various referrals I need going, I guess. Fuck. How do I tell everyone?

(Image: Steven Beatty)

A small note which was documenting a massive moment in time.

Paper Journaling

Journaling into a physical notebook can be very gratifying. There's something about that connection between pen and paper that's peaceful, and some would say missing if you use a smartphone app. I find the convenience of a phone, and its ease of backing up data to be enough for me.

The real benefit of journaling with paper is that it can provide you with more room to be creative. You can hand draw pictures and use coloured inks. Many smartphone applications have tried to emulate the experience of pen and paper, but they're not quite there yet.

Video Journaling

Another format that is great for journaling and documenting your life is video journaling.

There are many options for recording yourself on video that can be as private or public as you like.

I tried recording some videos using YouTube, but it wasn't for me. I find the written word and photos to be more of a comfortable format for me.

Why Journal?

Writing your thoughts down into a journal can be very therapeutic, as I mentioned at the beginning of this chapter.

Why is that?

Writing down words, and looking at them there in front of you, gives them a sense of *realness*. A feeling that you are releasing them out of your head and that the thoughts they represent, do in fact exist in the real world.

Sometimes, those of us in the in-between years may have thoughts that we are not prepared to share with anyone (even though maybe we should). Writing them down in a journal provides us with a way to get them out of our head, look at them, and perhaps reflect on them in a new way.

When companies are brainstorming ideas for their business plans, as an example, what do they do? They have meetings, and there's always someone standing in front of a whiteboard with a dry-erase marker writing things down. Seeing the words on the board stimulates new ideas, and before you know it, they've got mind-maps and outlines for the "next big thing." They've identified possible hurdles to reaching their goals and, they leave that meeting knowing what the following steps are going to be.

Without writing things down, they very well may have spent the whole meeting doing nothing more than just eating donuts. Now, I'm the first to enjoy a donut, but nothing productive was done.

You can do the same thing with journaling. Get those thoughts and concerns and fears out of your head and see where it takes you.

Chapter 18
Planning Ahead

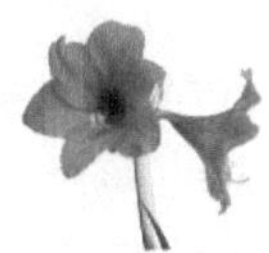

Planning for a future decline in health and eventual death is something everyone should be doing, not only those of us with Huntington's disease.

We're all aware of the uncomfortable fact of life that death can happen at any moment. We've all heard the cliché:

> "You could get hit by a bus tomorrow, so enjoy every minute."

Or something like that.

It's true we could. The purpose of this book is to be a handbook for Huntington's disease in-betweeners, but as I said, *everyone* should be getting their legal affairs in order. Hopefully well before they're hit by that bus at 106-years-old or becoming symptomatic for HD and losing the cognitive capacity to do so.

I discussed caregiver burnout in a previous chapter. It can be a difficult task for caregivers to make decisions on behalf of their loved ones if they're not feeling completely sure that they know what their loved one's wishes were.

Take the time to sit down with your partner or loved ones today and start the discussion. Not just for the in-betweener, but have the discussion *both* ways. Your caregiver and possible future decision maker need to make *you aware of their* wishes as well. As I've said already, *everyone* should be planning for their future decline in health as soon as able. Even if you don't have the funds to pay a lawyer to make everything legally binding, starting with the discussion can be so helpful for future decision makers.

Below are some topics for discussion to get you started. Before moving on, however, please remember that I am not a lawyer and laws can vary from nation to nation. If you are looking for specific legal advice, reach out to a law professional. Ultimately, you will need a lawyer to put your decisions on paper and make them legally binding, but as I said, start with the discussion.

Advanced Directives

Advanced directives, or advanced care planning, is about coming up with a plan *now* about how you wish to be cared for in the *future*. It's about deciding who you would like to act on your behalf if you're no longer capable of making decisions yourself. It's about ensuring that your wishes are understood and clear to all even though you may no longer be able to voice them.

Planning like this is great for everyone involved. You'll know that your wishes are understood. Your decision-makers and healthcare practitioners will feel as though they are doing what you would want, especially in an emergency.

This planning gives everybody peace of mind.

As I mentioned previously, the first step in advanced planning is sitting down with whoever it is that may become your decision-maker in the future and ensure that they know what it is you want. What do you want to happen if your heart stops? Where do you want to live? How do you want your care to be undertaken? What kind of treatments would you want or not want?

Think about what *you* find important and have a discussion.

After deciding on a person, or people, to be your substitute decision-maker, ensure that they understand what that role means and entails. They need to be agreeable and available to act as your representative for future decisions.

For the decision-makers to be legally able to act on your behalf, they need to be appointed as a Power of Attorney for Personal Care.

Speaking to a lawyer to ensure that everything is being done adequately is vital. The terms I've mentioned above may be different in your area-of the world, but there will undoubtedly be a legal process for you to assign a decision-maker.

Insurance

Obtaining additional insurance may be something you'll want to consider during the in-between years as you plan. Life insurance is a typical example.

For many in-betweeners, the thought of leaving family behind at a relatively young age can be quite concerning and stressful. Possessing additional insurance if you're able to, can help to ease that stress and provide some further security for the family as they move forward in life.

Speaking with a knowledgeable insurance broker can be very useful here as many people have no clue where to start when it comes to insurance.

Bucket List

Merriam-Webster defines "bucket list" like this:

> "A list of things that one has not done before but wants to do before dying. From the phrase kick the bucket (to die)."

Part of planning for the future involves attempting to limit regrets. It's impossible to eliminate all regrets, of course, but taking steps to minimize them can go a long way when it comes to acceptance at the end of life period.

Now, I'm still feeling confident that an effective treatment for slowing the progress of Huntington's disease is not too far away. Although that may be the case, everyone should have a "bucket list" of sorts, even if they're 100% healthy.

Remember, Mr. Bus.

My list is not very long. Some trips. Taking the kids on a Disney Cruise, that sort of thing, but it's there.

What's going on yours?

Brain Donation

An important part of Huntington's disease research is studying brain tissue. This process is more straightforward of course, following a person's death.

I know I'm not interested in sharing any brain tissue right now. I need every cell I can get!

There are "brain banks" in many developed countries that accept brain and tissue donation from Huntington's disease affected individuals.

Planning is critical to ensure the process runs smoothly and efficiently. As you can imagine, it can be quite the undertaking to have your brain removed following your death and shipped across the country, but wow, what an adventure for your brain!

I make light of the topic, but as with any other form of organ donation, the process is a well-oiled machine that runs smoothly behind the scenes. Planning for brain donation can ensure that all goes well at the time of death and the caregivers are not running around at a difficult time trying to make arrangements16.

Following the Latest Developments in Huntington's Disease News

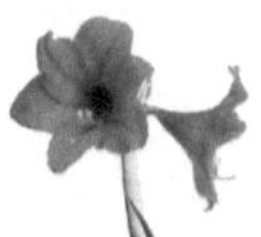

The internet is a big place, and I mean *big*.

It can be a scary place as well if you're not sure where to go to obtain information, especially as it relates to your health. Searching for Huntington's disease information on a site like YouTube as an example can lead you down a frightening road of videos with titles such as "*the top 10 worst diseases ever known to man!*"

There are methods for obtaining accurate and trustworthy information on Huntington's disease, however, and some of them are *even* on the internet.

HD Buzz

Since 2009, HD Buzz2 has been the number one trusted source for Huntington's disease news, specifically with a focus on the latest in HD research and study.

The site is run by Dr. Ed Wild and Dr. Jeff Carroll, who have unarguably become celebrities in the HD community around the world. They present Huntington's disease news and information in a jargon-free manner with extra injections of humour.

Dr. Wild is a Neurologist based in the United Kingdom. Dr. Carroll is an American professor who not only studies Huntington's disease, he also carries the gene mutation himself and is an in-betweener like us.

The reason I mentioned previously that HD Buzz is the number one source for Huntington's disease-related news is twofold.

Firstly, whenever there is an HD related press release from a drug company as an example, perhaps about some new breakthrough in Huntington's disease research, HD Buzz will take their time and review what is being put forward.

When they write about the news, they are sincere and forthright and will let those of us in the HD community know if this news is something to get excited about or not. They will let us know what the report may mean for future HD studies and remove all the "spin" from the press release.

Secondly, Dr. Wild and Dr. Carroll are very involved in the world's Huntington's disease communities and frequently travel to conferences and events to speak.

The HD Buzz content is translated into numerous languages, covering the world over. Also, all the HD Buzz subject matter is shared with a "creative commons licence." This means that it can be shared anywhere.

If you ever get a chance to hear Dr. Wild and Dr. Carroll speak, I highly recommend it. Their positivity and hope for the future are infectious.

Facebook Groups

The fantastic thing about the rise of the internet is how it has provided an outlet for like-minded people to interact and learn from each other.

This can be either a positive or a negative thing depending on the situation. In the case of Huntington's disease, which as we know is entirely a rare condition, the internet can provide a way to interact with other in-betweeners that we likely wouldn't have otherwise met.

Facebook is the social network that immediately comes to mind. Our mothers are on it. Our grandmothers are on it. Your cousin's friend's sister's nephew is on it.

And, there's a whole lot of in-betweeners on it.

Facebook has something called "groups" which are essentially chat rooms created by a user with a specific topic in mind. Groups can be private or public, and some require that you be approved by the group's creator before you can post and participate in the chat.

Chat is great, but the other salient feature of Facebook groups is the sharing of articles and information. Like minded people can share a news piece they have found exciting, and it's a great way to learn new things about whatever it is that interests you.

Of course, the information seen on Facebook should be read and reflected on with a critical eye, as there is the risk that it may not be entirely accurate.

I've seen, on more than one occasion, a piece of Huntington's disease-related news sweep across social media like a tidal wave. Only to find out (usually once HD Buzz had a chance to review it) that it was not a trustworthy piece of news.

With that word of caution, however, if you're a Facebook user, dropping in on a Huntington's disease-related group can be useful time spent.

Association Newsletters and Chapter Meetings

Becoming involved with a Huntington's disease Association is a topic I discussed in depth in chapter five of this book, but I thought it would be worth including here as well.

Associations are an excellent source of HD news and information. This news is dished out in a variety of ways, from newsletters to emails to social media. You can obtain information by attending a chapter meeting, or you can maintain some privacy and stick to the other means of accessing your Huntington's disease news.

Chapter 20

Is Huntington's Disease Predictive Testing Even Worth the Trouble?

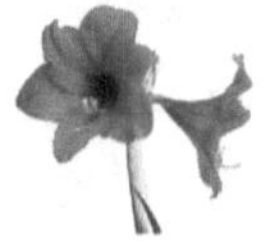

To Test, or Not to Test?

To undergo Huntington's disease predictive testing, or not to undergo Huntington's disease predictive testing? That is the question.

And, I have no answer.

That's because there is no easy answer. No one response would be appropriate for everyone. Deciding to move forward with the genetic test is an *extremely* personal decision.

And, every at-risk HD family member is different. Some will get tested as soon as they can, while others will never get tested.

Don't Rush into the Decision

If you are still in the decision phase of your thinking about Huntington's disease predictive testing, do not rush. You might want to rush, but don't do it. Take your time.

Access and take advantage of the genetic counselling that comes along with the testing process in most places. Spend a lot of time thinking about a lot of questions and *write those questions down*. Bring that list to the counsellor and then spend some more time thinking following that.

If you have a spouse or partner, involve them heavily in the process. Have them write a list of *their* questions and concerns as well. Allowing them to feel comfortable sharing their thoughts is vital.

Once You Know, You Can't Un-Know

Once the cat is out of the bag, so to speak, you can't put it back in. It's a silly cliché, but appropriate. Once you know your Huntington's disease genetic status, you know. It's part of your medical record. Most developed nations have laws in place to protect you from genetic discrimination, as I mentioned in chapter eleven of this book, but there it is. Out of the bag.

Keep in mind that if you do turn out to be carrying the mutation, know that there is a great deal of support out there. Even if you're feeling very alone, you're not.

I'll repeat it. *You are not alone*!

There are in-betweeners everywhere who are just like you. Experiencing the same fears and anxieties. Asking the same questions about planning for the future. Symptom seeking at every turn.

Reach out to your local Huntington's disease Association. The support available from them for those of us in the in-between years is invaluable.

Do I Have Any Regrets?

I'm the type of person who wanted to know my genetic status as soon as I realized I might be at risk. I think a lot of that had to do with my age at the time of 40-years-old.

I already had a family and a stable career. I had a pension and life insurance, and I had no concerns about genetic discrimination. If I was in my twenties and just starting out in life, my decision to be tested might have been different.

In my line of thinking, not knowing my HD genetic mutation status would add more weight to my wheelbarrow of worry. I would still be symptom seeking and wondering about every little trip and stumble, but on top of that, I would constantly be wondering about the status of my Huntington's disease overall. I'd be asking myself,

"Am I putting myself through all this worry for no reason?"

So, no, I have no regrets. For me, undergoing the predictive testing was worth the trouble.

Chapter 21

When Symptoms Start

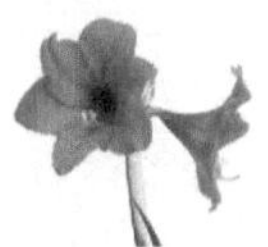

Being an in-betweener can be tough, there's no doubt about that. Many of us find ourselves symptom seeking from time-to-time, but how do we know that symptoms *have* actually started?

That's a very complicated question. Firstly, it's important to understand what is even meant by "symptoms starting."

What does it mean to be symptomatic?

Traditionally, Huntington's disease was said to be in the symptomatic stage when motor signs of the condition had begun, such as chorea. It's now commonly accepted, however, that HD is more complex than that and is not solely just a motor disease.

As pre-symptomatic in-betweeners, we are said to be in the pre-manifest period of our Huntington's disease journey. This phase continues until we slide through a prodromal period which is defined by the: "development of subjective symptoms or objective neurologic abnormalities1."

Now, this move from the premanifest period into the prodromal period is not a clear boundary that is crossed overnight. It's likely a very gradual process.

"It is increasingly agreed that a 'prodrome,' often lasting many years, of symptoms, signs, and subclinical abnormalities frequently precedes the emergence of more evident disease features1."

Moreover, it's agreed that as an in-betweener approaches the symptomatic period of their Huntington's disease, they often lose the ability to demonstrate insight into their signs of HD.

As an in-betweener myself, this aspect of the disease frustrates me to no end. The thought that this illness can sneak up on me and take over my life while I live in complete ignorance of it is something I find infuriating.

- What if I'm messing up at work and don't even know it?

- What if I'm an asshole at home and I don't see that?

The literature seems to reveal that this lack of insight is more commonly directed towards motor signs, rather than cognitive or behavioural:

"Some HD expansion carriers have clear motor abnormalities but report no symptoms; more commonly, subjective complaints of cognitive and affective symptoms precede motor onset1."

But, that doesn't provide me with a whole lot of comfort. I still worry a great deal about losing an understanding into my cognitive and behavioural stability, even though I know my loved ones are keeping a close eye on me.

"Thus, though a relatively distinctive prodrome of cognitive, motor, and neuropsychiatric dysfunctions clearly exists in most patients before formal motor onset, the fact remains that in an individual case, it is by definition impossible to diagnose prodromal HD 'beyond reasonable doubt.'1"

So, as you can tell, knowing when early signs and symptoms of Huntington's disease begin to occur, or when we have entered that prodromal period, is difficult. It's often a gradual process over years until we reach the point where a Neurologist can formally diagnose that we are in the early stage of HD.

> "The early stage of HD is a time when symptoms, signs, and most important, the ability to function in everyday life can change rapidly and be challenging for patients, caregivers, and health care professionals."

From that point on, we are no longer in-betweeners. We have moved into the symptomatic years. It's a horrible and frightening thought. Keep your head up.

An effective treatment will come.

What do we do if we think we're symptomatic?

If you think you're having early prodromal symptoms, such as difficulty concentrating or managing your affairs, firstly, talk to a friend or loved one. No one knows you better than a spouse or a parent or a close friend.

Have a conversation with them and see what their thoughts are. Trust that they are being honest with you and not trying to hide things from you. If they respond with,

> "What are you talking about? I haven't noticed anything."

Take some comfort in that.

Secondly, write the symptom or concern down, perhaps in your journal. Keep a list. If you have falls, make a note of each fall and where it occurred. Bring that list with you to your next Neurologist appointment. If your next appointment is seven months away, don't hesitate to make an early appointment to discuss your concerns. The Neurologist can provide you with so much piece-of-mind if they tell you they don't see anything concerning.

And, if they do see something of note, they are there to support you with managing whatever sign or symptom you may be experiencing. Remember, although there is no treatment for Huntington's disease in general, there are treatments to help with specific symptoms.

If you are beginning the symptomatic phase of Huntington's disease, there is a great deal of support available for you and your loved ones. Reach out to your local HD Association. Access counselling. Hug your friends and family every day. Email me: stevenmbeatty@gmail.com.

Chapter 22

I Look Forward to the Day When There Won't be a Need for this Book

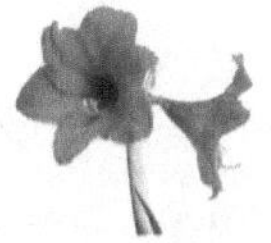

I had initially entitled this chapter: **I hope that one day there won't be a need for this book**. I read that and thought, "good grief, why am I using the word *'hope'*!"

Of course, there won't be a need for this book one day because science *will* conquer Huntington's disease! I have *no* doubt. When will that be? I have *no* idea. But, as with the onset of symptoms in HD, I believe it will occur gradually over time.

I once heard Dr. Jeff Carroll, from HD Buzz, speak at an event and a question came up asking when a cure may be a reality. He replied, and I'm paraphrasing here, so the words are not precise:

"I see a day where there is a treatment for HD that will delay the age of onset of the disease by a little bit. Then, not long after that, another therapy will come along that will delay it even longer. I see a bunch of little treatment milestones that will eventually delay the age of HD onset more and more, to the point where we can all die of old age before we die of Huntington's disease."

It was a brilliant statement and places everything into perspective. Sure, there may be one ground-breaking treatment that cures the disease altogether. What a day *that* would be! But, it's more likely that we will take baby steps.

One treatment option works its way through the scientific process and results in effective treatment. Not a cure, but something that delays the onset of our symptoms by five or ten years. Then, another treatment option works its way down the pipeline and delays the HD for another ten years.

The next thing you know, we're able to hold off the onset of Huntington's disease indefinitely. Maybe even with a once-daily pill.

I can dream, can't I?

As that all becomes a reality, you can throw away this book because we'll all be happy, non-symptomatic in-betweeners until we die at 108-years-old, like everyone else.

Chapter 23

Calls to Action and Conclusion

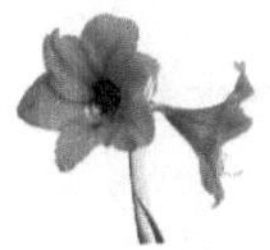

"It's not the result we were hoping for."

Everyone has a story. A struggle. Huntington's disease is mine and if you're reading this book, perhaps yours as well.

When you're faced with a struggle, there are two things you can do:

- Roll over and let it control you, or

- Accept it and take control.

Let's take control. All of us in-betweeners, let's do it. Remember, knowledge is power, and together we just learned a bunch.

We learned some Huntington's disease basics, such as CAG re-peat scores and genetics. We discussed caregiver burnout and anger. We touched on fear, guilt and symptom-seeking. We started thinking about the future and talked about family planning.

This book was put together to act as a handbook for Huntington's disease. Specifically, for those of us in the in-between years, but applicable to caregivers and families as well.

Here are some calls to action for you to take away

Huntington's disease is a very complicated subject, and it can be hard to keep up with all the latest news. There are always new things to learn and further research studies being released. Keep your eyes on HD Buzz. As I mentioned in a previous chapter, it is the number one source for trustworthy Huntington's disease information on the internet.

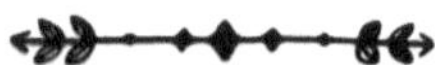

Consider reaching out to other members of the HD community, either through social media or Associations. I understand it can be a challenging thing to do and experiencing concern about genetic discrimination is understandable as well.

With that said, interacting with other in-betweeners can be so therapeutic. Why? Because you realize you're not alone. You see real faces. You have real conversations. That can go a long way in helping your overall sense of well-being.

If you're considering becoming involved in research, firstly, on behalf of all in-betweeners, *thank you*. Personally, I think anyone who participates in research on behalf of a group or population of people, to be a hero. Plain and simple.

Secondly, start with Enroll-HD. Having your data in the Enroll-HD database will open you up to many other studies as they come along as it's now common for scientists to recruit study participants directly from the Enroll-HD system.

Also, Enroll-HD is non-invasive, meaning, you're not being stuck with needles or taking any experimental medications. It's an easy start to being a research subject. With that said, part of the Enroll-HD process is running through some cognitive testing and word recall exercises. Don't fret; everybody comes out of those exercises thinking they did awful and must be symptomatic for Huntington's disease!

One more thing about Enroll-HD. They also recruit non-HD family members to act as control subjects, so grab your spouse or a sibling and make a day of it. My wife and I both take the day off work for our annual Enroll-HD appointment and turn it into a "date day."

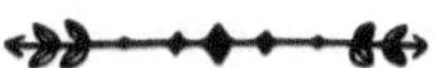

Think about planning for the future and getting all those legal affairs in order. Talk with your loved ones about what *your* wishes are if the time comes that health decisions about you need to be made and you're no longer capable of doing so yourself.

Advanced planning is not a task that's unique to Huntington's disease positive individuals, and it should be undertaken by everyone. So, while you're telling your partner about your wishes, make sure they are making theirs known as well.

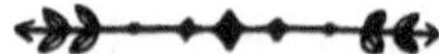

Exercise, exercise and exercise some more. Remember, research suggests that there may be a link between regular exercise and delaying symptom onset in Huntington's disease.

More research needs to be done to strengthen this conclusion, but exercise is good for us anyway, so what the heck! Aim for thirty minutes of good aerobic exercise every day.

If you're feeling angry, talk to someone. Remember our cheesy cliché: *"anger is one letter away from danger."* Talk to your spouse or a loved one. Chances are, if you've been demonstrating a lot of anger lately, they are aware of it and would be happy to talk about it.

Speak with your Neurologist about the anger. There are treatments to help keep it under control, including counselling and medication. This goes for other mental health issues as well, such as depression and suicidal ideation.

Don't wait. Stop reading this and talk to someone right away.

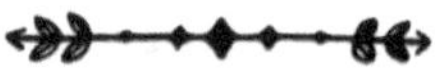

Symptom-seeking is something all in-betweeners do from time-to-time, but try not to get lost in it and miss a whole weekend.

If you find yourself stuck in a symptom-seeking rut, where you are spending a great deal of time thinking about something, acknowledge what you are doing and put that thought in your pocket. Don't judge yourself for the symptom-seeking.

Move your focus to the moment you are in and be mindful. Mindfulness is defined as:

"A state of active, open attention on the present. When you're mindful, you carefully observe your thoughts and feelings without judging them good or bad. Instead of letting your life pass you by, mindfulness means living in the moment and awakening to your current experience, rather than dwelling on the past or anticipating the future."

Mindfulness and meditation can be very helpful when it comes to maintaining our sense of overall well-being and keeping our head from getting lost in those feelings of anger, depression and symptom-seeking. There are many books on the topic, as well as classes and retreats to participate in, so have a look around and consider learning more about it.

Thank You

From my family to yours. Thank you for reading. Good luck in your battle, my fellow Huntington's disease warriors.

(Image: Steven Beatty)

About the Author

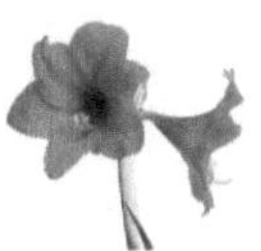

Steven Beatty is married with two kids and lives in central Ontario, Canada. He works as a Registered Nurse in the home care sector assisting members of his community with accessing home support services, making the transition into long-term care, and navigating an, often complex, health care system. He possesses a Bachelor of Science in Nursing Degree from the University of Victoria.

Steve is part of a Huntington's disease family himself and received a positive result on his HD predictive genetic testing in 2015. Since that time, he has developed a passion directed at advocating for the Huntington's disease community and has been hard at work forming a Huntington Society of Canada Chapter in his, somewhat remote, home area.

As a wannabe guitar hero, Steve is sad every day that he doesn't have the patience to actually learn any songs. Steve would also benefit from some more exercise and a tad less time spent staring into his smartphone, but those are stories for another day.